Time Flies When You're Alive

OBIT

LINKE, Francesca Draper. Songwriter, composer died at her home after a long battle with cancer on March 27, 1986 at age 37. Born in New York City, daughter of portrait artist William F. Draper and Barbara Cagiati Draper. Wife of actor Paul Linke, mother of Jasper, Ryan and Rose. Sister of William F. Draper, Jr. and Maggie Draper. A private memorial service will be held in the garden of her home in Mar Vista on April 13, 1986 at 3 P.M.

Time Flies
When You're Alive

A Real-life Love Story

Paul Linke

A Birch Lane Press Book
Published by Carol Publishing Group

A Birch Lane Press Book
Published by Carol Publishing Group
Birch Lane is a registered trademark of Carol Communications, Inc.
Editorial Offices: 600 Madison Avenue, New York, N.Y. 10022
Sales and Distribution Offices: 120 Enterprise Avenue, Secaucus, N.J. 07094
In Canada: Canadian Manda Group, P.O. Box 920, Station U, Toronto, Ontario M8Z 5P9
Queries regarding rights and permissions should be addressed to Carol Publishing Group, 600 Madison Avenue, New York, N.Y. 10022
Carol Publishing Group books are available at special discounts for bulk purchases, for sales promotions, fund raising, or educational purposes. Special editions can be created to specifications. For details, contact Special Sales Department, Carol Publishing Group, 120 Enterprise Avenue, Secaucus, N.J. 07094

Manufactured in the United States of America
10 9 8 7 6 5 4 3 2 1

Library of Congress Catologing-in-Publication Data

Linke, Paul.
    Time flies when you're alive : a love story / by Paul Linke.
    p.   ;   cm.
    "A Birch Lane Press book."
    ISBN 1-55972-183-9
    1. Draper, Francesca—Health.   2. Linke, Paul.   3. Breast—Cancer—
Patients—United States—Biography.   I. Title.
RC280.B8D735 1993
362.1'9699449'0092—dc20
[B]   92-37589
                                                                                                CIP

Preface

One month after Francesca's memorial, a director-friend, Mark W. Travis, suggested that I create a one-man theatrical evening based on the eulogy which I had delivered. Inspired by its message, he felt others could benefit as well.

I considered the idea for almost a year before I began to work on the play. I decided that my purpose was twofold: first, the work would serve as a catharsis; second, I wanted to bring death out of the closet.

We live in a culture where sexual partners freely discuss their desires. Yet death remains taboo—untouched and denied. We do not deal with it. We walk around convinced that it is going to happen to everyone but ourselves. As a culture, we celebrate birth, but resist and deny death.

Having participated in three home births and one home death, I learned that these experiences share a common bond and are in many ways the same. They are both part of the natural order of life and serve as our connection to a higher power and to life itself.

I have come to recognize the preciousness of our time on earth, and to embrace each day as the gift it truly is. Many people spend their moments as penuriously as a miser holds on to a dollar. *Is our glass half empty or half full?* I've come to the conclusion that our great fear of dying creates tremendous feelings of isolation and is a source of difficulties among people.

I've developed something that I call the Pit Boss Theory of Life, which is the notion that God has dealt each of us our respective hands which we play. Like any good card player, we all have been taught to hold our hands close to our chests so people can't see our cards.

My theory is that if at any moment in our life, we could be the ultimate pit boss, the man or woman who walks above on the catwalk and looks down on all the hands that are being played in the casino of life, we would see that we are all playing the same hand. I decided to risk showing my hand in the belief that you would recognize yours in mine.

We live in fiercely competitive times, where everything has been turned into a contest of winning or losing. This is even true in the arena of illness, where recovery is equated with success and dying denotes failure. We all cling to this life on earth as if this is what it's all about. Perhaps, as Steve Levine says in *Who Dies?*, "survival is highly overrated." Death is the natural resolution of life. Let's not allow our fear of death to keep us from living.

Incredibly, my theatrical catharsis was a tremendous success and continues to have a life of its own. During the past five years, I have performed my one-man show all over the United States, as well as in Europe. *Time Flies* was filmed as an HBO feature presentation. Ironically, what began as a healing for me has become a healing for millions. However far-reaching its effect has been, it all comes back to Francesca. She taught me and her loved ones so many things. Through *Time Flies When You're Alive* she continues to provide lessons for us all. It is my love song to her.

Acknowledgment

Nanci Linke-Ellis was an invaluable ally in bringing this book to life. A gifted screenwriter, Nanci has selflessly contributed countless hours at the computer and generously lent her talents to this project. There is no way I can ever thank her enough for her efforts, insight, and willingness to keep me moving forward. We fought, laughed, and sipped cappuccinos while reliving these experiences together. Without her help, support, and love, there would be no book. Nanci is also my younger sister.

I want to thank the following people who have been a great support to me and my children.

Edie Appleton, Scott Belyea, David Brubaker, Bill Bruns, Warren Christensen, Pam Danzig, Susan Dietz, Bobsey Draper, Jane Dystel, June and Paul Ebensteiner, Robert Egan, Steve Ellis, Steve Friedman, Donna Gaffney, Elizabeth Forsythe Hailey, Kendall Hailey, Christine Healy, Dave and Nancy Garden, Mary Jane Horton, Life on the Water, Richard O. Linke, Karl Johan Ljungberg, Michael Mann, Patrician McCarthy, American Michael, National Hospice Organization, the O'Briens, Laura Owens, Dennis "Little Guy" Redfield, John Ritter, Nancy Morgan Ritter, Mark W. Travis, Marion Rosenberg, Majid Roshangar, Alton Walpole, and Walter Ward.

Thanks to Jane Reed for the pencil sketch.

I would like to express special thanks to Ed Victor, who promised me he'd sell this book.

Very special thanks to Hillel Black, who was greatly moved by my one-man show and had the insight to buy the book. His wisdom and guidance have been invaluable to me. I also enjoyed our lunch at the zoo in Central Park.

And thanks to Denise O'Sullivan, who edited the manuscript and believed in it and the importance of its message. Her charm, wit, and youthful exuberance helped propel me to its completion.

*This book is dedicated to
all those who are a part of this story . . .*

especially my children.

Time Flies When You're Alive

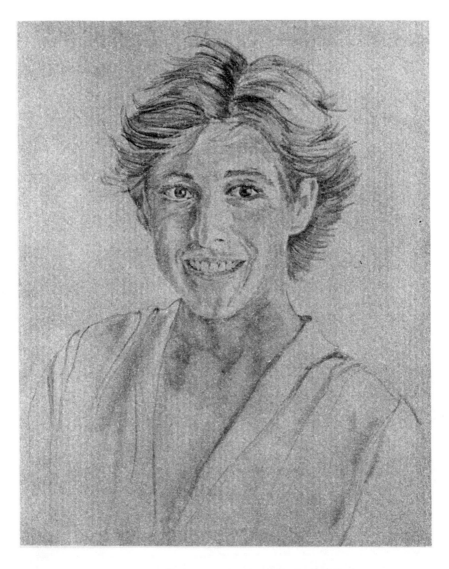

To CHEX- THE MOST VIBRANT BEING I KNOW —
MUCH LOVE, JAMES WANES
12/13/85

A Memorial for Francesca

"I'll love you forever... Thank you for my family."

On April 13, 1986, in the beautiful Brentwood garden of John and Nancy Ritter, 250 people gathered for Francesca's memorial. Everybody took their places on stark white chairs on an immaculately groomed lawn while I assumed my position at the podium to deliver the eulogy. Francesca had made me promise that it wouldn't be a sad or mournful occasion. She wanted a party in her honor with food and booze, a "wham-bam down at the Ashram." Her wish was for us to celebrate her life and remember that she would live on in our hearts.

I'd thought long and hard about what I might say that would convey her wishes and, in my typical fashion, had written nothing down. There was an air of uncertainty as I stood and looked out on the loving faces gathered there.

I began, "I met my future in a doorway at a party in Laurel Canyon. She was a comet of light."

After five minutes, people began to laugh. By the time I had finished, twenty minutes later, the mournful emotions in the garden had been transformed into a joyous celebration.

I signaled my friend Joe Landon that I was ready, and he brought a single white helium balloon up to the podium and handed it to me. I turned my back on the group and released it. As the speck of white rose up into the clear blue cloudless sky, I shouted, "I'll love you forever, Chex!"

1

After a few moments, Joe then handed me four white helium balloons with their strings tied and knotted together. I released them and said, "Thank you for my family." As the balloons began their widely divergent journeys, I turned back to the gathering and signaled that the ceremony was over.

The guests stood and slowly dispersed. Some went for the food and drinks, others lingered to gaze at the disappearing balloons while many simply stood and held one another.

I glanced at the children who were running freely on the periphery, and my eyes stopped at the sight of a floral arrangement sent by my dear friend Julie. In the center of the display were two sterling roses, the same flower worn by Francesca and me at our wedding. I realized that our love had reached its fullest bloom at the moment of her death. I searched the sky one last time for her balloon and thought back over our ten years together, our marriage, three home births, breast cancer, home death and life.

Love had led us through the valley of her death and enabled us to overcome her fear of abandonment and my fear of commitment. Together we had learned one of life's greatest lessons. Time flies when you're alive.

The Last Waltz

"Can I give you a hug?"
"If you want to."

I met my future in a doorway at a party in Laurel Canyon, a tiny quasi-community nestled in the Hollywood Hills that is known as a haven for artists such as Joni Mitchell, Frank Zappa, and Jack Nicholson. My invitation to destiny happened on November 20, 1976. It was a classic fall Saturday in Los Angeles. I was home watching the traditional big game between my alma mater, USC, and our bitter crosstown rival, UCLA.

Once the game ended with another USC victory, I hopped into the shower to get ready to attend a party that evening. At this point in my life, I was an actor between jobs and a single man between romantic liaisons. My first live-in romance had ended the previous year and its length suggested that I still hadn't conquered my two-year relationship syndrome.

No matter who my girlfriend was, everything would always be great during the first year—a lot of laughs, late meals. She would even let me watch sports. But once we reached the one-year point, difficulties would arise, leading to the inevitable breakup. I always placed the burden of blame on the woman.

When my first live-in girlfriend moved out, I started to take early-morning walks through the canyon to deal with the pain of our breakup and to reflect on my other prior relationships. I began to understand that I was at least 50 percent of the problem, that when things would get too intense, I would shut down like an off-line nuclear reactor. It was at this point that I swore to myself that the very next time I met a significant other, I would break through this barrier and clear the way for intimacy by confronting my fear of commitment.

3

The opportunity greeted me when Francesca came through a doorway. Her eyes were indelibly blue. They reminded me of the clear blue lakes in Switzerland.

"Are you from Switzerland?" I asked. She laughed and said, "No. But my family used to ski at Gstaad on spring break."

She smiled and I was dazzled. Impulsively, I pleaded, "Can I give you a hug?" She ambivalently responded, "If you want to." Tentatively, I put my arms around her. She was a passive participant in our embrace. Even though a little voice in my head told me to stay away, I invited her to attend the "Last Waltz" concert with me in San Francisco. She politely turned me down, but before the party was over, Francesca admitted that she wanted to get to know me and asked that I call her.

Five days later I was at Winterland, a San Francisco concert hall, to attend the Last Waltz, the final public performance by The Band. It was a grand Thanksgiving Day affair produced by the late concert promoter Bill Graham. He created an event that began at 4:00 P.M. with a complete turkey dinner. Afterward, a full symphony orchestra, framed by the backdrop used in the *Gone With the Wind* ballroom scene, played a series of waltzes. It was an incredibly romantic sight to watch the lovely-looking people float around the dance floor. A beautiful raven-haired woman in a black beaded brocade evening gown approached and asked me to dance. I was in heaven as we swirled around the dance floor for what was to be my own Last Waltz.

The concert was without a doubt an event in which the sum was truly greater than each of its magical parts. It was a night to remember.

As the evening unfolded, The Band played one song after another with amazing passion and urgency. They were joined by assorted friends and artists who had either influenced or been influenced by them.

By the time The Band played "The Night They Drove Old Dixie Down," the room was on fire. Van Morrison danced an

Irish jig and sang "Caravan" as he hopped across the stage on one leg. I felt as if we could all go no higher. Later, Eric Clapton played guitar with Robbie Robertson, who gestured to Eric as if to say, "Take it, take it." An apparently reluctant Eric stepped downstage into the spotlight and blistered a guitar riff that was straight from God. By the time he had finished, I felt as if my consciousness had been stretched from corner to corner of the hall. I was as high as I could be. The energy was thermonuclear.

At that instant, an incredible wave of music emanated from backstage. Like a supernova, Bob Dylan shot up a ramp and took center stage. Wearing a wide-brimmed hat and a white bandanna, he sang "Baby Let Me Follow You Down" and then broke into "Forever Young." A verse in the song hit directly home to me:

> May your hands always be busy
> And your feet always be swift
> May you have a firm foundation
> When the winds of changes shift
> May you build a ladder to the stars
> And climb on every rung
> But may you stay forever young.

My heart exploded and I realized at that moment, a whole era in my life was ending. The 1960s were finally over—even if it had taken until 1976. Bob Dylan had given us all a message: Close this chapter of life and move forward, always keeping the joy of youth within our hearts.

With that mandate, I thought of Francesca's beautiful blue eyes and saw in them a clear vision of our lives merging. By the time I climbed back into my old yellow Dodge van, I was determined to pursue Francesca Draper and marry her. My heart was full as I drove south. It seemed as if life was a wide-open highway.

Paul/Chex Mate

"I, Francesca, take you..."
"I, Paul, take you Francesca..."

As soon as I returned to Los Angeles, I called Francesca and made a date to take her to an L.A. Rams game. She seemed enthusiastic, but later admitted she had thought we were going to a *baseball* game. We decided to extend our first date by going to see *King Kong*. Later we munched on a Caesar salad, and by the time the evening was over, it was obvious that our feelings were mutual and that we would have a future. It wasn't long before we started to spend all of our time together.

We were both flower children of the sixties, but we had come from vastly different backgrounds. Francesca had been a New York debutante. Her parents, both artists, were divorced. Her father, William Draper, is a renowned portrait artist whose works hang in museums like the Smithsonian and the National Portrait Gallery. Chex (a nickname imparted by her brother, Willy, probably over a bowl of cereal) and her family lived on Manhattan's Upper East Side and spent summers in the Hamptons. She was a classically trained pianist who preferred to perform her own musical compositions. After graduating from Sarah Lawrence College, she left New York in pursuit of alternative lifestyles. Chex moved to the mountains of Colorado and became a brown-rice-eating vegetarian, a candlemaker, and an antiques store owner. She continued to play music in the Boulder area and came west to L.A. to further her musical career.

7

The Linkes were an entirely different story. Even though I was born in New York, all of my formative years were spent in southern California. I had been reared in a show business family, and my parents too were divorced. My mother, Maggie, was a former Richard Hudnut twin, a housewife, and a devoted mother to me and my sister, Nanci. My father, Richard O. Linke, a well-known television producer and personal manager, had exposed me to a high-spending, free-wheeling lifestyle. He pressed me to study law, but I chose to go into acting. I was trained in theater at the University of Southern California, where I obtained both my undergraduate and graduate degrees. Like Francesca, I had ultimately rejected my parents' lifestyle to "do my own thing."

The first time we made love was December 12, 1976, under the sheets of my king-sized water bed in the double garage apartment up in Laurel Canyon after a Robin Williamson concert. It was so sweet and her body seemed so vulnerable. As she climaxed, I had the image of sparkling spring water gushing from Mother Earth. She was my "clear light" lover, my New Age main squeeze.

I felt so lucky and she was so beautiful. It was around 3:00 A.M. when she said, "Paul, do you realize what we just did? When we made love like that, do you realize that we created a bubble of light that surrounds us and binds us together. If we are faithful and only make love to each other, the more energy we'll create, the more light we'll fuse into our bubble, the more luminescence we'll give off, and the more we'll be bound together."

Even though I didn't fully grasp the metaphysical concept, her "Lover's prayer" became our code of behavior. I believed in the importance of fidelity and feared that if I was ever unfaithful, our "bubble" would rupture.

I had never felt so deeply about anyone. I had found love and was already envisioning us as husband and wife. We spent all of our nights together and began to operate as a couple. We threw dinner parties to meet each other's friends. This was a new experience for me, and I worked very hard at our relationship. After my last failed romance, I had vowed that when I met my next "significant other," I would push through my two-year barrier and not shut down; I would say the hard things and do my best to keep communications on-line. I would go for it, commit, and make it work. With Chex, it all seemed so easy.

They were the best of times. Francesca and I walked the beaches, sipped café au laits, and made love on a foam pad in her funky Venice loft. It was the first time in my life that I looked into a woman's eyes while making love to say from my heart, "I love you." I had never used those words during sex before, but with Chex those big little words were as much a part of the experience as the physical release.

A year passed and it was time to meet her mother. I can still remember the first time I saw Barbara Draper. She came down the stairs of the Venice loft and I joked, "Is that a Cagiati I see?" The invocation of her maiden name totally cracked her up, and we immediately became friends. Francesca and I threw a sit-down Thanksgiving dinner for forty people in her honor. We whipped up a major feast out of Francesca's tiny, boatlike kitchen. Later, over pumpkin pie and cognac, Barbara and I had a warm conversation. We were off to a great start.

The day after Thanksgiving, however, Barbara took me aside and asked me about my intentions. She was worried about her daughter and wanted me to make up my mind about our future.

"If you want to get married," she said, "you should start thinking about it. I'm going to take her away to the desert for a few days and I'd like you to use the time to come to a decision."

It was the push that I needed. I feared that Barbara would take her back to New York and find her an eligible bachelor. Recognizing that I didn't want to lose her, I decided I wanted to get married and bought her an engagement ring as a Christmas present.

There are two things in life that I know I do well. Talk. And give gifts. In the true Richard O. Linke tradition, I decided to have a little fun with the presentation. I bought an ironing board, wrapped it in a big box, and told Francesca that it was her "big gift." Underneath the tree, however, was the diamond ring, wrapped in a small box.

On Christmas Day, she excitedly opened the box with the ironing board and politely thanked me. She did a pretty good job of hiding her feelings. I felt bad because I knew she was upset, but I still didn't let on about her real gift.

As the day went on, her spirits sank and the ring box still lay hidden under the tree unopened. Finally I couldn't stand it any longer and said, "Oh, I forgot to give you this little present."

When she opened the box, I asked her to marry me. She burst into tears and admitted how upset she was over the ironing board.

We decided on an October wedding, and plans were put into motion. We decided to live in her Venice loft, so I gave up my Laurel Canyon apartment and moved in with my two dogs, a rocking chair, my record collection, and an antique queen-sized oak bed.

As soon as everything was in place, my two-year-relationship syndrome reared its ugly head. I had assumed that true love was a low-maintenance affair that required no extra effort. But as soon as we entered the second year of being together, we began to take each other for granted. Lust never lasts, and I eventually had to confront the fact that there is no such thing as "happily ever after." The endless afternoons of bliss ended. Doubts seeped into my subconscious. Looking back, I wonder if the problem was my upcoming commitment, or if it was just the Yasir Arafat Terrorist Life Principle—when things are going good and you least expect it, someone is going to blow up the whole scene.

As the wedding got closer, the feelings intensified. Even though I had privately sworn to hang in there and keep the relationship on track, I struggled and became depressed. I couldn't hide my feelings from her because we had always told each other the truth. I told Chex how I felt, and this put a lot of pressure on her. Our wedding was only six weeks away.

Actually, we were both freaked out. She went to psychics, had our tarot cards read, and prayed. I woke up in the middle of the night and drank Jack Daniel's. I lost weight and became so depressed and frightened that I didn't think I could go through with it. It was a tough time in our lives.

We didn't tell anyone about our troubles. Chex felt that if others knew about our problems, their focus of attention would "concretize" the situation. She believed it was up to us to solve it. She reminded me that I chose her in a clear state of heart and mind and said that marriage was a serious challenge. This was just the first test.

And so we clung and hung in there until finally the week of our wedding arrived. We had decided to get married on the beach of Paradise Cove, a beautiful inlet just up the coast from Malibu. We asked the Reverend Jim Conn from the Church in Ocean Park to perform the ceremony. We felt it was important that the wedding reflect our personalities, so we asked him to help us write our vows.

To make it a festive and theatrical event, I hired a brass quartet to play music as the guests assembled on the sand. Francesca and I wanted to demarcate the place of our commit-ment and went to meet with Anders Holmquist, a flag maker. Anders, a tall, lanky Swede, was intrigued by our idea of a wedding flag. He gave us each a color test and analyzed us by our choices. I was very nervous that he would take one look at our selections and regretfully inform us that we clashed.

But he didn't. We talked about the design, and he came up with the concept of a star for me, the actor, with a heart over it to symbolize our love. Francesca threw the I Ching and came up with her "chord," a musically notated spiritual statement. When we were finished talking about the design, I inquired as to the cost. I almost passed out when he said it would run about $350. I had no idea that it would be so expensive. I thought about reneging on the deal, but felt obligated after all the time he'd spent with us. As Chex and I walked out, I whispered, "I never knew there was so much money in flag-making."

No matter how much attention you give to the details, there's always something that gets overlooked. In my case, it was the World Series. When we set the October 14 wedding date, I didn't even consider the possibility of a series between the Los Angeles Dodgers and the New York Yankees. It was a beautiful time of year for a wedding, but not if you were an obsessive, lifelong Yankee fan.

The Yankees had got into the series by winning a playoff game against the Boston Red Sox. Yankee shortstop Buck Dent hit a high fly ball into the screen above the green monster in Fenway Park and broke Boston's heart. I grew up on Yankee baseball, and this was the most exciting moment I had ever experienced as a fan. I literally jumped up in front of my television and screamed as the ball left the yard.

Another ingredient in the emotional prewedding stew was the fact that it was a week of absolute "CHiPs" madness. I was in my second season portraying Highway Patrolman Artie Grossman on the NBC series, which starred Erik Estrada and Larry Wilcox.

Five days before the wedding, we were filming way out in the San Fernando Valley on an unopened section of the 210 freeway that the show always used. The script that week called for a stunt involving an ambulance with a baby in it and an overturned tractor-trailer. For five days, I reported to location at 7:00 A.M., sat in my tiny mobile dressing room, and waited. Each twelve-hour day passed without my being called before the camera.

The stunt took four days to be completed. I still had so much to do for the wedding, but I couldn't leave. With each hour that I didn't work, my frustrations grew. I felt as if I wanted to smash the mirror in my honey-wagon dressing room or break something to release the tension, but I just sat there and fumed.

I had tickets to Game 1, but I couldn't go because of my "CHiPs" schedule. I tore up the tickets as the 5:00 P.M. starting time passed and barely made it home to see the last couple of outs. Bob Welch struck out Reggie Jackson in one of the most exciting "at bats" I'd ever watched.

I also had tickets to Game 2, but I gave them away because my dad and his second wife were coming to dinner to meet Francesca's parents. After my parents divorced in 1972, my father promptly married a Las Vegas show girl named Bettina. She was 6'2" and the absolute fantasy of his life. They had three kids and lived a rather glamorous lifestyle. They were meeting the Drapers, who had also divorced around the same time but had remained friends.

Francesca and I were nervous about how comfortable my dad and Bettina would feel in our funky abode. We didn't have matching plates, silverware, or wineglasses. Francesca and I didn't even have a table large enough to seat everyone, so we pulled two tables of different heights together. It turned out to be a fun night, and everyone got along fine.

The next night, a travel day for the Yankees and the Dodgers, Rev. Jim Conn came to make sure that we were both okay. I was still fighting my demons when Jim arrived. The mood passed, however, once we cracked open a bottle of chardonnay that I had bought for the occasion. Sometimes I think that my wedding came down to that one bottle of wine. As soon as we drank and talked, I felt better. The wedding was on.

October 13, 1978—Friday the thirteenth. Another Yankee-Dodger travel day. My mother hosted our rehearsal dinner at the Chronicle restaurant in Santa Monica. I planned the menu of Caesar salad, duck, wild rice, and creamed spinach. It was a fantastic sit-down dinner for fifty people, filled with joyful toasts and good wishes.

Francesca and I felt it was very important to do the traditional thing of not sleeping together the night before our wedding. I went to the Miramar Hotel, where my family was staying, while she went home with all her women friends. My male friends threw me what was probably the most boring bachelor party of all time. All we did was sit around and talk while Chex and her entourage went through their sisterhood ritual. Rites of passage surrounded, enveloped, and entrenched us.

October 14, 1978—Our wedding day and Game 3. Ironically, I had an early-morning callback for a 7-Up commercial. I figured what the hell, and went to it. After all, how often do you get married and have a commercial callback on the same day? I got the job, but they never made the spot.

The day began as an overcast, ugly kind of day, but at 3:00 P.M., when it was time for us to gather on the beach at Paradise Cove, the clouds parted and the sun broke through.

The flag was perfect. It rippled in the breeze while everyone gathered round for the nuptials. The brass quartet played as Bill escorted his daughter down the cliffside path to where I stood barefoot on the sand in my new three-piece suit. As I watched her move toward me, I was certain in my heart that I was doing the right thing. I was thrilled to take her for my wife. And the bride wore...shoes.

We stood under our flag emblazoned with the music clef, the star, and the heart, and recited our carefully written vows:

> I, Francesca, take you, Paul,
> to be my husband
> I, Paul, take you, Francesca,
> to be my wife

I will share my life openly with you
And speak the truth to you with love
I will honor and care for and love you
With tenderness and affection
And I will cherish and encourage
Your fulfillment as an Individual

I will live and evolve
In faith and in hope
And with love
I will nourish our Union
Throughout all the changes of our Lives.

It was only later that we came to understand the ultimate meaning of those words. We were children of the sixties becoming adults in the seventies, making promises that would be sorely tested in the eighties.

Home Care Primer

"I don't understand...like surgery is no big deal."

M y first glimpse at Francesca's intimate relationship with her own body, and how it affected her attitude toward the medical profession, occurred just prior to our belated Hawaiian honeymoon. Chex had been experiencing pelvic pain, so I nervously called one of my father's country club doctor-friends. He ran some tests and came back with the diagnosis of an ovarian cyst. He recommended surgery as soon as possible, which prompted a freaked-out Francesca to ask a million questions (I was never one to ask a doctor *any* questions). He patiently assured us that the operation could wait until we returned home from our trip to Hawaii.

By the time we got home from the doctor's, Francesca was furious. She fumed over the doctor's cavalier attitude toward the surgery.

"I don't understand him. He acts like surgery is no big deal. Of course, it's not happening to him. If it's not important enough to operate right away, how can it be important enough to operate at all?"

Chex decided to research ovarian cysts in *Back to Eden*, her bible on herbal medicine, and found a natural course of treatment to cure her condition. This was the first time I had ever seen her in action. She used herbs and douches, adhered to a specific diet, and drank teas. She sat in the garden with her robe open and exposed her abdomen to sunlight, which she filtered through a rose-colored glass plate.

Part of me thought she was absolutely out of her mind, but another part was fascinated by her commitment to and faith in these unorthodox methods.

By the time she went to see the doctor for a follow-up visit, the cyst had vanished. He was a specialist in the field and could not explain how it had happened. He was amazed, since he had fully expected to perform an operation.

This success was a source of great pride for her, and it had a profound effect on me. I had watched her tap into a very strong spirituality and generate incredible healing powers over her own body. It made me believe in her.

Home Birth

*"He's a great-looking baby boy...but...isn't he a
little blue?"*

C hex informed me that we were pregnant and due in early
March. She proudly smiled and said, "I hope you know
we're having this baby at home." I thought I had grown as a man,
but this little bombshell freaked me out. I didn't even know that
people still did that.

"There's no way we're having this baby at home, Francesca.
You've got to be out of your mind. We are having *our* baby in a
hospital where it is safe."

She calmly looked at me and said, "Paul, having a baby is not
a disease. It is the most perfectly natural thing that a woman
does."

I had a major dilemma on my hands. Francesca had a very
strong point of view about birthing; maybe it was time for me to
open up my own limited intellectual vocabulary to understand
what this perspective of hers was all about.

We went to the L.A. Childbirth Center, where we met with
midwife Vi Barone. We spoke to people who had gone through
home delivery. I came to understand that, in childbirth, I was
only the coach. It was my responsibility to be there for her, rub
her back, and give her ice chips when her mouth got dry. I
would be her emotional support and keep track of her contractions. But the fact was, when push came to shove, it was Francesca
who was having the baby.

Birthing is a very personal experience, and it is a woman's right to choose whatever environment suits her. If she wants to have it at home, great, or at the hospital, so be it. Even if she decides to have it at the Sizzler, by the salad bar, it is her right to choose!

We enrolled in classes at the childbirth center taught by Tandy Parks. Each week, we took our pillows and gathered in her home, watched slide shows, saw demonstrations, and listened to discussions. One week, as we were all getting to leave, Tandy announced, "Next week we will discuss circumcision."

I froze. The thought had never occurred to me that we would have a boy. I just assumed we would have a girl. Don't ask me why. We had already picked out the name Rose, but had no name for a boy. Now I had to deal with *this*. Did I want my son circumcised? I wished I hadn't been. Why cut off all those nerve endings that feel so good? We don't live in barbaric times anymore. We have hot water and soap.

So I did my research. I began by talking to pediatricians. Next thing you know, I was talking to everyone I knew. Are you circumcised? Have you ever slept with a circumcised man? Have you ever slept with an uncircumcised male? Which do you prefer? Who do you think enjoyed it more? If you had it to do over...? You would have thought I was doing an update for the Kinsey Report.

I was confused. I had no idea what to do. My friend Dennis Redfield provided the most interesting argument for circumcision. He was going to have his son circumcised because he felt that some day, when they took a shower together, his son could look at him and not feel different or alienated.

Pregnancy agreed with us. It was the first time in our marriage that we didn't have to think about birth control. I mean, we had obviously failed. It was a really great time. As Francesca's due date grew closer, I began to get nervous about having sex with

20

her. I couldn't shake the image of my penis poking the baby in the head, which made Chex laugh.

Every afternoon, she would go out to her garden for a combined digging and "squatting" session. She explained it was to strengthen the muscles she would need to push the baby out. This practice continued until the birth. She was committed to breast feeding and prepared for it by rubbing her nipples with a rough washcloth in the shower. She took good care of herself and watched her diet. She was a Warrior Woman, physically fit, well schooled, and emotionally prepared to take responsibility for her experience.

Valentine's Day—February 14, 1980. We celebrated the Day of Hearts over a beautiful Italian meal and went home to watch the Winter Olympics. The downhill skiing competition excited Francesca, an avid skier. We watched an Austrian make an incredible run that put him in first place. During a commercial, Francesca got up and headed to the bathroom. I heard a loud "pop" and realized that Francesca was the source of the noise. I turned and saw her standing in the middle of the room, with water flooding out from beneath her terry cloth robe. It looked as if a five-gallon bottle of spring water had been overturned.

All I could think about was getting to the phone. As I walked through our kitchen, everything seemed to be in slow motion. I reached Tandy, childbirth instructor and labor sitter, who came right over. She wryly confirmed my suspicions that Chex was indeed in labor and went to call the midwife. We were in the midst of a major rainstorm, one of the most intense in my thirty years in southern California. Vi finally arrived in a torrential downpour. She clutched her satchel beneath her little umbrella as she approached our house on the dark Venice street. Her shadowy figure bore an eerie resemblance to the *Exorcist* poster.

She checked Francesca and told us we still had a long way to go. She wasn't dilated. It was just early labor. We wondered if a mistake had been made on the dates, because the baby still wasn't due for nearly a month. Vi reassured me that one month either way was fairly common and said that the size of the baby's head and abdomen indicated it was full-term.

Meanwhile, Francesca got down to the business of labor, using the Bradley method of breathing. It involves deep breathing versus the rapid panting of Lamaze. I sat back and recorded contractions. Every time Francesca had a contraction, I would note the time and the length. She would contract, I would write the information on a piece of paper. This went on for *four* days. By then, I was either underwater or over my head, depending upon which analogy you prefer. The point is, I had so many different contractions written down on so many separate pieces of paper all over the house that I didn't even know what contraction went with which day. I was beginning to lose it.

I left to take a short walk and when I returned some fifteen minutes later, Chex had gone through "transition" and was now in hard labor. To me it all looked hard. Seven P.M. And as they used to say on "Miami Vice," "it was going down now." Vi was amazing. Her hands reminded me of Keith Jarrett, the pianist, and the flourishes and quickness with which he played his improvisational pieces. She worked with alacrity and effortless grace with Francesca, who was immersed in this Bottom Line Woman Ritual. I was overtaken by the notion of what home birth represented for Francesca. She insisted upon taking responsibility for her own experience and wanted the freedom to make choices. She did not want to be strapped down to a hospital gurney attached to a fetal monitor. And most of all, she did not want to be tempted with access to drugs. She wanted firsthand experience of the ring of fire (not the Johnny Cash song, either), the moment during birth when the baby's head fully crowns and a woman's vagina is stretched to its maximum.

Her reasons for desiring this undiluted experience were not masochistic. She truly believed that only by living through this moment could a woman experience the flush of ecstasy that comes at the instant the baby's head is born. To Francesca, it was the moment in a woman's life where she was most in touch with her own "womanness."

At 7:18 P.M., the baby was out. *He* was born. He was laid on Francesca's tummy while the cord, still purple and pulsating, came out from between her legs. She glowed with ecstasy; I felt as if I had just been run over by a Mack truck. I now had a son, a little boy with a little penis dangling in the air. I knew by looking at him that I was never going to circumcise this kid. If God made him this way, there was no way that I was going to go "chop chop."

We put the baby on the breast to get him to try suckling. I glanced at Vi and noticed her concerned expression. The baby was still blue, but I knew he would remain that way until he took his first "breath of life." I waited and remembered our child-birth classes. Francesca and I had been obsessed by the possibility of newborn breathing difficulties. Tandy had always said, "Paul, we've talked about this before. Both midwives have oxygen tanks in the trunks of their cars. In over three hundred births, we've only had to use the oxygen *two* times. Relax."

But here we were in our Venice loft home. Our baby was out, he was blue, and he was *not* breathing. As Vi's concern grew, she tapped him on the back and vigorously massaged his chest. She reached into her weathered black satchel and pulled out a blue bulb syringe and began to suction out his mouth and nose. None of her attempts to start him breathing worked. The kid was stone blue. I tried not to add any bad vibes to the situation.

"Gee, Vi," I said. "He's a great-looking baby boy...but...isn't he a little blue?"

Vi turned to Tandy and said, "You'd better go get the oxygen."

I sat there thinking how ironic it was. Our worst fears had come true. Here we were doing the most natural thing a woman does, the midwives had done it over three hundred times, and only needed the oxygen *three* times now! So much for the best-laid plans.

The oxygen was wheeled into the house. It looked like a two-wheeled golf cart people use to pull their clubs. As I watched Tandy, our oxygen golfer, the phone rang. Francesca's father was calling from New York. Isn't is amazing how some people always have the worst telephone timing?

During this moment of absolute chaos and fear, I learned one of life's important lessons. If you do a home birth, *turn on your answering machine!* I didn't want to hurt his feelings, nor did I want to alarm him, but what could I say? "The baby's out, he's blue. I'll get back to you."

We spoke briefly and I told him that everything was okay, but I couldn't really talk. As I hung up, I turned my attentions back to Francesca, who was extremely anxious about the baby. The oxygen tube was put under the little baby's nose and he started to turn pink. As he began to breathe, all the tension in the room gradually dissipated and was replaced by a warm wash of joy. Francesca burst into tears of relief at the sight of our firstborn. The baby was put back on her breast to get him to suckle. Vi clamped the cord in two places and I cut it. I looked at my wife and child and was chilled by the realization of the enormity of the responsibility that I had taken on.

I knew about "father bonding" from the one book that I had read. So with that idea in mind, I took off my shirt and placed my newborn son against my naked chest, hoping he'd remember me when he was a teenager. He's twelve now and it's worked so far.

I was fascinated by the birth of the placenta, which we then placed in the special metal bowl saved for this purpose. We were going to plant it in the backyard beneath a rosebush. Francesca had read in a journal that if you ate a tiny piece, it would help stop the bleeding. Later, she and several of the women present ate a sliver. I graciously passed. I thought about it, but just couldn't do it. I don't even like sushi.

About an hour after the baby was born, Francesca noticed that the little guy was experiencing a shortness of breath and seemed very uncomfortable. Vi checked him and decided to call the pediatrician. Once a baby is born, its well-being becomes the responsibility of a pediatrician. He directed us to meet him with the baby at UCLA Medical Center. Francesca was totally spent from four days of birthing and was unable to go to the hospital. Thankfully, Vi offered to accompany me.

So there we were, loading the baby into the Peugeot. We drove over to UCLA Medical Center on a rain-slick night. From the freeway overpass, we could see the colored lights reflecting off the wet sheen of the pavement. As I drove, I looked at Vi holding my newborn baby and puzzled over the paradox. We had prepared for and successfully achieved a home birth, and yet I was now delivering our unnamed baby to the hospital.

As we approached UCLA Medical Center, Vi held the baby and I stepped on the rubber mat that opened the automatic doors. A pretty blond candy striper-type named Terry first looked at me and then at Vi before saying, "Are you the mom?" The fact that Vi was in her middle fifties made me question whether this young woman was capable of caring for my child. Before I had a chance to answer my own question, the baby was taken away while I filled out some forms. Forty-five minutes later, I was finally escorted to the neonatal clinic, where the baby had been taken. His arrival could have been premature, which would have explained his breathing difficulties. The doctor told me, "Mr. Linke, we started your son on antibiotics about ten minutes ago."

"Why?"

"Well, Mr. Linke, he was born at *home*. In about an hour, we're going to have to do a spinal tap."

"What are you talking about?" I asked.

"Well, Mr. Linke, since so much time elapsed between the breakage of the water and the actual time of delivery, there is a two percent chance your son might be septic. You wouldn't want to take that risk, would you?"

I looked at the baby, who lay naked on a metal table behind double panes of glass. He was being probed by doctors he didn't know. He was crying hysterically and I couldn't comfort him. I had brought him here for their help and this was their call, their territory.

It was about one-thirty in the morning when Vi and I drove back home. I crept into our darkened Venice loft and walked up the twelve wooden stairs just in time to see Francesca's silhouette stagger out from behind the bamboo curtain in the bathroom. I flicked on the light and saw she was shivering in a cold sweat. She was hemorrhaging heavily because she didn't have a baby to suckle on her. She collapsed into bed and fell into a deep sleep as I lay down with her.

At 3:00 A.M. I was still awake and staring out into the darkness. I listened to the silence and thought how weird it all was. It was so quiet. We delivered a baby at home that night, but we were still all alone.

Name Game

"How could you not name him?"
"Dad...we've got a name."

The day after our baby was born, Francesca remained exhausted. I went to visit the baby. But first I had to find an electric breast pump to help Francesca prepare to nurse. I obtained one through the La Leche League. As I walked into the woman's house, I mused over my first real responsibility as a dad. I had entered a whole new world. She was a nice woman who asked questions about the birth while she nursed her own rather large child. The baby was about three and obviously had never missed a meal. As a matter of fact, our conversation was continuously interrupted by the hungry child who climbed onto her mother's lap, yanked her blouse down, pulled her breast out, and tried to "do lunch."

I had never seen a child nursing before, much less a sixty-five-pounder. The kid was huge. I thought, "Oh, my God, is this going to happen to us? What are we getting into? Is our son going to nurse until he's eleven? Is Chex going to become a Slurpee machine?"

I rented the breast pump and took it home along with the woman's offer of help. While Chex worked on creating milk, I went off to UCLA Medical Center to visit our still nameless son, Baby Boy Linke.

I entered the neonatal clinic, a high-tech place where you had to scrub down and don a gown, cap, gloves, and mask to visit your child. Our newborn son was the picture of robust health compared to all the other preemies who struggled to survive. At six pounds ten ounces, he looked like the heavyweight champion of the world.

Baby Boy Linke's "next door neighbor" was so tiny that his skin was translucent and you could see the circulatory system at work. IV jars were jury-rigged to nurture the preemies toward life. In this high-tech atmosphere, our boy's breathing had normalized. He now looked totally fit. He wasn't in an incubator; he just lay there, totally happy with an IV in his ankle. I sat next to his crib, held his hand and sang, "Nobody does it better, nobody does it half as good as you, baby, baby, baby you're the best."

By the next day, Francesca was ready for a visit. We arrived with some breast milk that Chex had produced. She was totally horrified that they were feeding the baby sugar water. She had vowed that her children would never have sugar. Ironically, to this very day, my first son remains the ultimate sugar freak in our household.

We were told that he was being given sunlamp treatments because he was a little jaundiced and his bilirubin count was up. (Bilirubin is the orange-colored or yellowish pigment found in bile, blood, urine, and gallstone's.) Francesca argued, "Of course he's got a high bilirubin count. You've got him on incredibly powerful antibiotics and there's no fresh air in this place. What are you doing to his system?"

The hospital staff did not like the fact that the baby still had no name. Because he was born at home, they had nothing to do with the birth certificate that I had filled out.

Finally, we were told that if the baby's bilirubin count went over nineteen, the staff was going to give him a full blood transfusion. Francesca was beside herself when she told me,

"You and I will physically remove our baby from here if they try to do that, do you hear me? We will steal our child before we let them do that."

Finally, the bilirubin count decreased and we were able to take our child home. It was with great relief that we picked him up at UCLA, thanked everyone, and drove home. We were so excited to have our brand-new family under one roof.

We started our life as parents and quickly learned what no one ever tells you. *What do you do with it?* Our birth classes, prenatal and birthing books, and all of our exhaustive studies had only taken us as far as the moment of birth. Nothing prepares you for life with a child. There are no instructions on the back of a box. We were on our own.

During our first night together, the three of us slept in the same bed. I placed our son on my chest, and he promptly peed on me about three or four times. Francesca peacefully commented that she had read somewhere that it was a sign of acceptance.

Our baby still had no name, and we were still determined to find the *right* name. Whenever people congratulated us on his birth, they would immediately inquire, "What's his name?" My standard reply was to say we just didn't have one yet.

I never realized the political implications of the statement. You would have thought that I was telling people we were twisting the kid's toes with pliers or something. People were incensed.

"How can you do that to your child?"

"How could you not name him?"

"Don't you understand how important a name is?"

Francesca and I were adamant about not naming our child until we found one that we felt fit him. We read every name book we could find, including the *The New Age Pet Name Book*, which I guess is as California as you can get.

Six weeks later, we were finally up to the *J*'s, which were very big in the early eighties. Jason, Jordan, Jennifer, etc.

"How about Jasper?" I asked. It followed Jason. Chex and I both looked down at our baby boy and agreed, "That's it. Hi, Jasper."

I immediately called my father, who had really been on my case. "Dad, guess what? We've got a name."

"Thank God," he said. "What is it?"

"Jasper," I proudly replied. "Jasper Draper Linke."

There was a very long pause before he responded, "You mean I waited six fucking weeks for you to come up with Jasper?"

I'm glad that we waited as long as we did to find the right name. It really suits him.

Ryan's Song

"Jasper, look..."
"...my baby bruddah."

The discovery that a second little Linke was going to be added to the chain came as quite a shock to both of us. Francesca continued nursing Jasper during the pregnancy until she realized that in order for baby number two to receive her full juice, so to speak, Jasper had to be weaned. There was a point earlier when Jasper wanted to wean himself, but Francesca didn't want him to. She enjoyed her connection to him and loved the feeling created by the hormones that are released during nursing. She also believed that her milk was providing him with natural protection against disease.

Months later, when she needed to wean him, he resisted her attempts. We probably should have let him stop when he wanted to. We could have perhaps avoided the trauma of the "tit de passage."

We were once again committed to a home birth. There was never any question in our minds about it. Despite Jasper's hospitalization, our home birth experience had been great. We worked with Vi again, and the pregnancy went along uneventfully. As we got closer to the delivery, we were really excited and tried to prepare Jasper for the new addition.

We were convinced that this time we would have a girl, but we were armed with a name for either sex, just in case. If we had a girl, she would be Rose, after my paternal grandmother. If it were a boy, he would be Ryan, which was my mother's maiden name. He would have three last names: Ryan, Draper, and Linke.

We were lying on the water bed at midnight, April 27, 1982, when her water broke. Water on water. I immediately called the labor sitter, who came right over. This was an entirely different experience. The labor was fast and furious and took less than five hours from the time Chex's water broke to the moment that the midwife went home. Not only was the delivery a complete success, but it afforded me the opportunity to catch our second child. In the flush of ecstasy and the expulsion of the water, blood, and fluids, I performed my task like Johnny Bench. Fortunately, the pitch was right down the middle. I was shocked to see a little penis hanging in space. I thought, "My God, I have two sons!" I was totally unprepared. Looking back, I realize how ill-equipped I was to lose my illusion of control. I have a sister, she and me. That was our family, an older boy and a younger girl. I was sure that I would have the same. Well, that's not how it works in real life.

It was 5:00 A.M. when Vi went home, leaving the three of us in bed. All the noise woke Jasper, now two and a half years old, and he came into our room right after Ryan was born.

"Jasper, look, you have a baby brother," we told him. He left our room for a moment and came back with a gift for his newborn brother. It was a quilted crib guard with elephants sewn tail to trunk. Jasper was in a daze when he looked at the new baby for the first time and said, "This is for my baby bruddah."

Now we were really a family. Another one of those things they never tell you is that having a second child is not twice as hard — it's really sixteen times as hard. It's the first thing I tell people who are expecting a second child. I guess it's like the Richter earthquake scale. The magnitude of the event increases exponentially. After the first one, you think you've got it down. But when that second one appears, the balls are all in the air and the juggling requires a lot more skill.

Thank God, Ryan was such a good baby. Chex and I had exhausted all of our fatigue "dollars" on Jasper's infancy. Just like his arrival into the world, Ryan's early days were the exact opposite of Jasper's. He slept through the night, a content and peaceful baby. Jasper had cried incessantly for the tit, while Ryan was a peaceful, gentle force in our home. Ryan is very proud of the fact that he is the only child whom I was able to catch. Being the middle child, it is particularly important that he has that distinction. It may not be the reason that we share a love for sports, but it probably does explain our close bond.

Francesca's Final Performance

You and me are like a story
Moving on down that line

After two births and five years of motherhood, Francesca had begun to feel as if her performing career was over. With my encouragement, she mounted a weekend concert series at the Powerhouse Theater in Santa Monica, a theater that she and I had cofounded with our friend Ry Hay. It truly was a powerhouse that had originally been built in 1902 by Southern California Con Edison to provide electricity to the surrounding neighborhood and the famous Red Line Trolley. As artistic director, I raised the money and organized the productions; Ry designed the theater; and Francesca created the outer gardens where audiences congregated before and after shows.

On the afternoon of her opening night, we sat outside during a break from the final technical rehearsal and savored the moment under the gentle February sun. We were sipping our foamy café au laits from the Rose Café and speculating on the weekend's excitement when the phone rang. It was Francesca's mother, Bee Draper, calling from Manhattan with the disturbing news that she had just been diagnosed with breast cancer. Chex offered her mother words of comfort and solace and promised to join her in New York once the shows were over.

She broke her mother's news to me. A strong undercurrent of fear passed between us, which neither of us acknowledged.

You see, the irony here was that Francesca had a lump in her breast too. A growth that she had had for a very long time. Before you jump to any conclusions, I must paint another stroke in the picture. Francesca was still a nursing mother. I don't know how much you know about breast feeding, but Francesca had taught me that there was a lot more to it than meets the eye. I must confess to being the typical male who believed that the only elements involved were a hungry baby and a full tit. I'd always thought that you just slapped the kid on and BANG! it was an "instant meal." Faster than a microwave.

To help me understand what she was going through, Chex had given me *The Motherly Art of Breast Feeding.* I learned that nursing wasn't always such a simple procedure. Bleeding nipples, lumps, and clogged milk ducts were all very much a part of the process.

Her first growth occurred while she was nursing Jasper. Francesca's initial reaction was, of course, not to go to a doctor. She once again referred to *Back to Eden,* her bible of herbal remedies. The book's author, Jethro Kloss, prescribed comfrey and heat. Chex happened to have a comfrey plant in her garden. She picked fresh leaves and placed them on her naked breast under a steaming hot hydroculator. Within ten days, without antibiotics or other medical intervention, the lump disappeared. She nursed Jasper for twenty months without any other problems.

Chex developed another lump while nursing Ryan. Once again she employed her tried-and-true methods, but it was to no avail. No amount of comfrey, heat, or prayer would dissolve it. This lump was different. I believed she sensed it. Perhaps, subconsciously, her fate was clear.

Night after night, Francesca would stand in the dormer of our bedroom to examine herself. The image of her probing the breast backlit by moonlight streaming in through the garden window will remain forever etched in my mind. It was as if her fingertips knew braille, but she was blind to the truth of their touch.

I watched her balance the scale of anxiety night after night. I finally lost patience and roared, "If it worries you so much, Francesca, why don't you have it looked at?"

I tried joking about it and satirized her little nightly vigil, calling it the "lump shuffle." She laughed when I mimicked her by probing my own breast. But the fear remained.

She became engaged in the daily struggle to discover how fate and free will interacted. In retrospect, I wonder: Did she know? Did she see her path laid out before her? A psychic later told me that my wife had chosen to be reborn in order to give birth to our three children and provide her loved ones with a great lesson in life and love. While I'm not sure that he was right, it is interesting to note the depth of emotion that her passage has evoked and how far its effect has rippled.

She wrote a song during this time period. It is called "All I Could Do":

> You and me are like a story,
> Moving on down that line,
> Sometimes it gets so hard,
> It's all I can do to hold on to you,
> All I can do to hold on.
> You say it's okay, okay.
> It's all right.
> But it's all I can do.

Terms of Endearment

"Honey, is this us?... Is this what's going to happen?"

W hen "CHiPs" was canceled in 1983, I entered a new phase of my life, which I now refer to as the "Television Actor Post-Series Graveyard." It's the place where all those faces you know and love on TV go when their shows are axed. At least, a large percentage of them. There are those few legitimate television stars that go from show to show. But let's face it, most of us get recycled into other careers, like Eddie Haskell, who became a small-town cop.

I felt as if I had been put into the grave still kicking, looking up at the dirt being heaped upon me by the industry at large. I silently screamed, "I'm still young, I'm a character actor. I'm not even supposed to get work until I'm forty. Don't you understand, I have talent. I can do things you don't even know about!"

But no one cared, nor did anyone express any interest in me. I couldn't get a job, I couldn't get arrested. I was still getting money from residuals, but I saw problems ahead.

I would always get the strangest reaction from casting directors whenever I mentioned my work on "CHiPs." I thought it was an accomplishment, but soon learned there was a stigma attached to our show. "CHiPs" and "cancer" are words that became totally synonymous for me. Whenever I'd mention *either*, no one would know what to say!

You have to be very, very, very careful about what you pray for in this life. All those years as a struggling actor, I had prayed to

God for a hit television series that would last five years. If only I had the foresight to pray for a *quality* hit television series! But for one word, I could have been on "Hill Street Blues." I could have been a Steven Bochco discovery. But no, I was stuck in the cosmic overview of life as Artie Grossman, comic relief, fifth banana on "CHiPs." I struggled to come to terms with being in the valley of my professional life.

By some small miracle, *High Tide* came across my desk. It was a play by Seattle writer Gregory Hurst that had a great part for me. I believed that the role of Corky would allow me to stretch creatively and be seen in a whole new light by the industry. Corky was a Vietnam vet who had no friends. A compulsive eater and drug user, he was a totally blocked character who was warped by life. In the third act, all of Corky's suppressed rage erupts and he breaks down and cries. I was thrilled to have the opportunity for this kind of theatrical catharsis. I believed that I could effect such an emotional performance that I would turn my career around.

The biggest challenge in assuming the role was that I had to cry in an intimate environment. I couldn't fake it because the audience would only be three or four feet away from me. I worked diligently in getting the part together, but still hadn't figured out how to make myself cry on cue in each performance.

During the rehearsal period, Francesca and I went to see the film *Terms of Endearment.* I didn't know what it was about, only that it was a popular film. It was a pleasant story until Debra Winger's character discovered she had breast cancer and that the prognosis was bad. I elbowed by wife and whispered, "Honey, is this us? Is this our story? Is this what's going to happen?"

She snapped in reply, "Stop it, Paul, stop it. Don't you know thoughts are things?"

Later in the film, when Debra Winger's children came in to say good-bye to their dying mother, I was overwhelmed. I sobbed during the scene where she put on her makeup and tried to stay composed so that her little children wouldn't know what was about to happen. I thought about my own children. What if this was us? The actor part of me took over and recognized that my response to this scene was the key to my being able to break down and cry in *High Tide*. This was my motivation, and I knew it would work.

At rehearsal the next day, it worked like a charm. The mere thought of Debra Winger and those kids brought tears. Afterward, cast members, moved by what I had done, praised my work and predicted how wonderful my performance would be.

But when opening night arrived and I came to that moment, there were no tears. Nothing. I knew the critics were out there and felt my whole career was on the line. I panicked, not knowing what to do. As a last resort, I substituted Francesca and our kids, and still nothing happened. The pressure was just too great.

I now realize, as an actor, that the truth of the moment is the truth of the moment. An actor can only be where he is at any given time and that's the appropriate place for him or her to be, but that night I felt I had failed.

After the show, there was a big party at Papa Louie's on Main Street in Santa Monica. We sat in the dark and ate Buffalo-style chicken wings and pizza as we congratulated one another. My agent sat next to me and said with too much wine on his breath, "You just do this brilliant kind of work and I'll do the rest." I didn't hear from the guy again for six months.

The one lingering memory that I have of that night is a beaming Francesca standing outside the stage door waiting for me in her new white dress. She came up to hug me and told me how proud she was. She looked so beautiful.

Ben Casey Time

*"Paul, your wife has cancer. I'm going to have to remove
her left breast."*

Francesca's weekend concert series proved a rousing success.
It was a glorious time for her. A shining star on the Powerhouse stage, she performed to full houses, standing ovations,
and encores.

During her performance, Chex dedicated a song she had
written for Jasper when he was a baby. She introduced the song
to the audience by saying, "This is dedicated to my first son,
Jasper. And as I told everyone last night, I was going to dedicate
it to both of my boys, and say this was a song for my kids, but it
really isn't. It is a song for Jasper because he inspired it. Some-
day Ryan will get his song too."

> Get Down on Your Knees
> (Jasper's Song)
>
> You don't have to cry
> You just have to be released
> You just have to be released
> And sometimes you may wonder why
> There are things you cannot know
> You just have to grow
> And if you think the changes gonna go away
> You'd better get down on your knees

You better get down and pray
And you will know life
With all its beauty and its strife
And the arrow of love gonna pierce you
And the arrow of love gonna pierce you
And the arrow of love gonna pierce you
To the bone

And you will get down on your knees
'Cuz if you get down on your knees
The angel of love gonna fly beside you
The angel of love gonna guide you
The angel of love gonna guide you
Where you need to go

Today you are so small
Tomorrow you'll be tall
I pray that you grow strong
That you meet the storm head on
'Cuz the shadow of fear
Gonna whisper in your ear
'Cuz the shadow of fear
Gonna whisper
What you don't want to hear

And you will get down on your knees
'Cuz if you get down on your knees
The angel of love gonna fly beside you
The angel of love gonna guide you
The angel of love gonna guide you
Where you need to go
                              —Francesca Draper Linke, 1981

That was her final public performance.

Ryan never got his song.

Two days later, Francesca was on a plane to New York to help her mom through the surgery. Francesca was suddenly face-to-face with one of Manhattan's top-of-the-line breast surgeons. During her mother's preoperative visit, Chex could no longer contain the anxiety about her own growth. In a moment of absolute panic, she leaned over the doctor's desk, pulled up her blouse, and asked, "Would you look at my breast too?"

The doctor took a cursory look and referred her to a specialist in Beverly Hills. He implored her to seek immediate attention, saying he didn't like the looks of it.

Bee's surgery went ahead, and only a lumpectomy was necessary. This best-case scenario was due to her age, the lump's early detection and her speedy action. All these factors contributed to her uneventful recovery. She is presently in good health and enjoying her life in New Mexico.

Upon Chex's return from New York, she began a series of appointments with Dr. Mitchell Karlin, a renowned surgeon. She underwent a physical exam, a sonogram, and a mammogram and finally was scheduled to have an outpatient biopsy.

It was 8:00 A.M. when the Peugeot pulled out of the driveway and headed to Beverly Hills Medical Center. We waved good-bye to our sons, who were playing in front of the house with our housekeeper, Josita. We told them we were going to run some errands and promised to be back in a few hours.

At Beverly Hills Medical Center, we were directed to the outpatient surgery floor to check in and then escorted to one of those funny little doctor examination rooms. It was bare except for a vinyl padded table that folded at one end with a paper sheet that ran down the middle; there was a stool on one side and stainless steel shelves along one wall. A nurse came in, handed Francesca a pale green shmatteh, and instructed her to change. It was quite cold in that room, and Francesca was very upset. She complained about the indifferent attitude of the hospital personnel and their lack of sensitivity in leaving her to freeze.

As she shivered on the cold table, I pulled up the stool and tried to comfort her. "Chex, I'm so proud of you, honey. You're finally taking responsibility for this lump. It's going to be such a relief to get rid of all this fear you've been carrying around. Francesca, you are *not* the cancer type. You are going to be fine. I feel it in my bones."

Two attendants brought a gurney into the room. After she was transferred to it, Chex was wheeled down to surgery.

I walked alongside her until we reached the surgical area. I sat on one of those cushy imitation-leather-really-vinyl-type couches and read an esoteric magazine like *People* or *Time*. All of a sudden, the surgical doors swung open. It was Ben Casey time. Dr. Karlin strode out with a fierce determination that was evident with each step he took. As he pulled down his mask, his eyes found me and he quickly came over.

"Paul, it is what I was afraid of. Your wife has a very large malignancy very close to her chest wall. Would you tell me, why did she wait so long? What was she so frightened of? Well, I'm afraid it doesn't matter now. I want to check her into the hospital today. I'll let her rest for a couple days, but then I'm going to have to perform surgery. Paul, your wife has cancer. I'm going to have to remove her left breast."

I tried to absorb his words, but the room started to spin around me. He jolted me back to the moment by suggesting we go upstairs and comfort her. As we walked, I asked if Chex knew and he nodded yes. When we entered that same funny little doctor's examination room, Francesca was lying there in the pale green shmatteh on that vinyl padded table with that thin paper sheet and looked at me with bewilderment. "Can you believe this, Paul? Can you believe this?"

They checked her into Beverly Hills Medical Center, and two days later, Dr. Karlin performed a modified mastectomy on her left breast.

Chex had never liked her own breasts. She had always felt they were too flat and hated the way her nipples pointed downward. However, she greatly mourned the loss of her breast and often spoke of how it had helped feed her babies.

To Chemo or Not to Chemo

"If I take Cytoxan...I would be sterile."

Two days after her modified mastectomy, I sat with Chex in her Beverly Hills Medical Center room when Dr. Karlin came in to give us the biopsy results. He was happy to report that all of the lymph nodes had tested negative, indicating no evidence that the cancer had spread. He also told us to expect a visit from the head of oncology, who would come by to discuss adjuvant treatment.

The oncologist, whose name I don't recall, was an interesting cross between Marcus Welby and Ichabod Crane. He came into the room that Saturday morning, pulled a chair next to the bed, and said, "I've spoken to Dr. Karlin and reviewed the biopsy. I have to agree with him. Because of the size and nature of the tumor and the fact that it was so close to the chest wall, my professional opinion is that you need one year of chemotherapy and six months of radiation."

Francesca immediately jumped to the offensive. "Dr. Karlin just told us that my lymph nodes were clear," she responded.

His reply was clinical, professional. "That's true," he began. "However, the tumor was so deep that Dr. Karlin and I strongly believe that this course of treatment is your best chance for a complete recovery." He was not the warmest man in the world, but his concern seemed genuine.

Chex absorbed what the doctor said and spent a few minutes in contemplation before asking, "What do you know about what

49

Mishio Kushi is doing with macrobiotic eating for cancer?"

Puzzled, he reacted as if she were speaking a foreign language. "I'm afraid that I've never heard of Mishio Kushi," he thoughtfully replied.

The intensity behind her questions grew, her face was still and serious. "Well, what do you know about what the Symingtons are doing down in Texas with visualization for cancer?" she pressed while fidgeting with her wedding ring.

"I'm afraid I've never heard of them, either," the good doctor said.

Chex continued to cross-examine him. "Well, what exactly do you know about holistic approaches to cancer?"

"I'm afraid that I know very little about holistic approaches to cancer," he tersely replied.

I sat there quietly and observed the tension between the two of them. I had been taught to always follow a doctor's orders and was unprepared for her polemic response. My nature is to mediate, not to confront. However, as I sat in the now silent room, I sensed there was no middle ground.

The exasperated look that Chex threw me confirmed my instincts. She had nothing more to say to that doctor. We awkwardly made small talk until he finally got up and left.

As the door slowly swung shut behind him, she looked at me and said, "Goddamnit, that is so typical. I mean, here is a guy who is supposed to be a cancer expert, but he doesn't even know what's going on in his own field. Why should I listen to that man?"

The oncologist left a list of the three chemicals that would be used. They were Cytoxan, Methotrexate, and F-5U. Together they made up a powerful chemical cocktail that was crudely designed to inhibit the fast-growing cells' ability to replicate. Within twenty-four hours, Chex had studied up on the effects that these chemicals would have on her body. She was distressed by what her research revealed. None were designed to enhance the immune system.

"Paul, do you realize if I take Cytoxan, it could cause permanent... *permanent* kidney damage, permanent liver damage. I'll lose my hair. Do you realize I could go through premature menopause? I would be sterile."

What you need to understand about Francesca is that she was a gardener. She loved the earth and the things she knew how to make grow out of it—her fruits, her plants, her vegetables, and her flowers. Francesca's instinct was to work her magic using natural measures. If she walked out of our house early one morning and found that during the night some snails had trespassed into her garden and devastated a favorite Swiss chard plant, she wouldn't rush off to a hardware store and buy a pesticide to annihilate the snails. According to Francesca, if you put poison into the earth, you were effectively putting it into all of us through the earth's water system. To her, we were all connected to this earth and it was our job to protect it, not abuse it.

She solved her snail problem in her own unique way. She researched how cultures that didn't have access to pesticides dealt with these nasty pests. Night after night, she'd go out into our backyard with her flashlight. She would gather up these invaders as they made their way toward their dinner and would put them in a bucket. When she was done gathering them, she would smash them to death with a brick. Then she would take the broken snail body fragments and spread them all around her garden because a book had told her that the stink of the rotting snails would deter any future visits by any other snails. My wife was the Charles Bronson of organic gardeners.

Francesca's whole system of beliefs now faced its greatest test as she lay bandaged in her Beverly Hills Medical Center room. She looked at me and said, "Paul, how can I, who won't even put poison into a garden—how can I put this poison into my own body?"

Dr. Karlin gave Chex thirty days to decide on her course of treatment. She worked feverishly trying to figure out how to beat this disease. Determined to find a natural solution, Chex read, researched, and networked in search of an alternative method to the conventional chemical approach she had been offered.

Francesca's aversion to chemotherapy stemmed from the notion that God gave everyone an immune system to fight disease. She couldn't see taking chemicals that would, in effect, annihilate her immune system as a sane course of action. Instead she sought ways to bolster her immune system and purify her body as a means of defeating her physical enemy.

During this thirty-day period, we saw the surgeon frequently to have him check the wound, change the bandages, and remove the stitches. Dr. Karlin was gentle in the way he handled Chex and respectful whenever he inquired about her decision. To show my support, I went with her to every appointment and sat on a little stool in the corner of the examination room. I always looked straight down at a particular spot on the linoleum-tiled floor.

There is another aspect to mastectomy. When does the husband get to view the disfigurement? When does he share in that loss with his own eyes?

The day Francesca called our "unveiling" finally arrived. I was sitting in my usual position when I heard her voice. "Paul...come over here." I slowly rose and walked over to confront the results of her surgery. I smiled at her before I looked down at her wound.

It wasn't ugly and it wasn't a turnoff. Flat and smooth, except for the fold of the incision, it reminded me of her brother's chest. After she put on her shirt and left the room, Dr. Karlin cornered me.

"Well, Paul, what treatment is Francesca going to do?"

"Dr. Karlin," I hesitantly replied, "she's looking for a cancer clinic in Tijuana, Mexico."

Grabbing me by the arm, he held me firmly up against the doorjamb. The softness of his voice belied the extreme urgency of his words.

"Listen to me, Paul. I'm the surgeon, I was in there. And let me tell you, we're fighting to save Francesca's life. This is not a game," he pleaded with me. "I want her to do the chemotherapy. I want her to take these drugs. Do you hear me? She won't listen to me. I can't get through to her. So I've got to get through to you. I want you to go home and talk to her. I want you to get her to take these drugs. I want you to get her to do the chemotherapy."

I felt as if I had been split into two. One half of me viewed Dr. Mitchell Karlin as one of the greatest breast doctors in the United States. To me, he was the Mickey Mantle of breast surgeons. He was the man you wanted on your team if you were in this fight. In my heart, I knew he was telling me the truth. At least what he understood to be the truth.

The husband-to-Francesca part looked at this man, whom I greatly admired, and thought, "What are you talking about, get her to do the chemotherapy? Don't you understand this is her body we're talking about? She believes these drugs are poison and they're going to kill her. What am I supposed to do, anyway? Go home and slap her around a bit, like Ralph Kramden, and tell her HEY, LISTEN TO ME, YOU'RE GOING TO TAKE THESE DRUGS!"

I persuaded Francesca to get a second opinion from another oncologist. His name was Van Scoy Mosher. When we arrived for our appointment, we found a newborn baby with its parents in the waiting room. Watching the mother being led away to a side room for her chemo injection made Francesca panic. We had entered the cancer world, where people all around us were fighting for their lives.

Dr. Mosher was a pleasant surprise for us. He was a "hip" oncologist with long hair and good looks. There were crystals all around his office. He had a lava lamp and a definite New Age presence but he was an M.D. and one of the best.

After listening to us explain Francesca's situation, he responded, "Well, Dr. Karlin is a fantastic doctor and if he said she needs chemotherapy, I'm not going to sit here and tell you he's wrong. Let me talk to him about it."

He showed us charts on breast cancer survival rates after seven years. They were based on various levels of lymph node involvement, the different approaches to chemical therapy and radiation, and the percentages of potentially increased longevity. But all his charts were based on lymph node involvement. There was no category on the charts for patients with *zero* lymph node involvement. Mosher agreed that Chex was in a gray area, but felt he should talk to Dr. Karlin before giving us his opinion.

A few days later, Dr. Mosher called to inform us that he agreed with Dr. Karlin, but felt he could devise an acceptable schedule of treatment. Francesca didn't buy it at all. She was more determined than ever not to put any poison in her body. I saw it in her eyes and heard it in her voice. I wasn't about to fight her on it.

I must admit that during this thirty-day period, I was a very passive supporter. I realize that I experienced the initial stages of denial. My reluctance to jump in and read books, make phone calls, and help with research really irritated Francesca. Actually, it pissed her off. To me, it was her body and her decision. It frightened me too much to take responsibility for that decision.

The deadline approached rapidly and Chex went into a frenzy. One afternoon, while I was out of the house, a dear old friend of her mother's, a survivor of brain cancer, called to tell her about the Health and Life Clinic in Tijuana. She claimed that tumors had literally been flushed out of her system and spoke highly of the man who ran it, Dr. Gary Young. By the time Francesca hung up the phone, she had decided that this was God's way of guiding her in a healing direction.

When I returned home, she excitedly informed me that she had made a decision. She found a solution she could live with.

When she wanted to have our babies at home, I stood by that decision and I gained richly as a man for having participated in those experiences. Since she had made this very difficult, bottom-line decision about her own future physical well-being, I felt it was my job to stand up and support her belief system and her choice. Maybe I didn't believe in her methods, but I believed in her.

The Long, Winding, Alternative Road

"Chex, it's just a little blister."
"It's back, Paul... it's back."

April 25, 1984. We left our children in the care of our housekeeper and drove the Peugeot to our destination south of the border. I did not want to go to Mexico. Frankly, I never wanted to go to any part of Mexico, even for recreational purposes. Acapulco, Cancún, and Ixtapa held no allure for me. But there I was, driving to Tijuana, the "crown jewel" of Mexico.

On the three-hour drive down, we did not speak. We were just two heads in a car heading south. I was so angry. This was not what our life was supposed to be about. I wanted it all to just go away. If this was what she wanted, then I wanted her to get it over with so that we could get on with our lives again.

By the time we crossed the border, I was distraught. We had left the United States of America, home to the best doctors in the entire world, to go off on an uncertain quest. I could not understand how she believed this would be her road to health. Looking back on that journey, I realized she was just as scared as I was angry.

We took our final turn on a little dirt road that led to the entrance of the Health and Life Clinic. It looked like the Alamo. It was two stories high, with big iron gates and a roof made of broken shards of glass that were probably used as a security measure in order to keep banditos from mounting any sort of assault, I imagined.

57

We were warmly greeted by Willard, a seventy-year-old, tall, lanky Iowan type who immediately began to tell us about his wife, Lu, and her cancer history. He explained that when Lu did not respond to chemotherapy, her doctors gave up on her. As a last resort, Willard brought Lu down to see Gary. She began his program and was still doing fine two years later. Willard had stayed on to help Gary with his work.

Willard led us into the main building, where we then met Dr. Gary Young. Gary was very rural by nature; a dark-haired healthy-looking, energetic man in his late thirties. His open work shirt revealed a stocky, well-built physique. Gary was warm and affable, with a firm grip and a big square jaw. After we sat down, he asked Francesca for her hand. He took a little needle out of his drawer, removed its protective plastic cap, pierced her finger, and squeezed out a drop of blood. Once it came to the surface, he reached back into his drawer and took out a glass slide and stained it with blood. He then took the slide over to a microscope behind his desk and flicked on the light. He examined the specimen and after a few seconds said, "Uh-huh, I can see the cancer right there."

I thought to myself, "You've got to be kidding me." To Gary, I said, "Can you really tell if a person has cancer from a drop of blood?"

"Oh, yes," Dr. Young said, "they've been doing it in Germany for over forty years."

"Would you like to be tested?" he asked.

Now, talk about a place to put a skeptic! There are very few words as paralyzing in life as "I'm afraid you have cancer." If someone diagnoses you with cancer, you'd better really believe that he knows what he's talking about.

"No, no, no thank you. I don't think I want to be tested. Maybe some other time," I quickly responded.

Dr. Gary Young's program included fasting, fasting, and more fasting. Hot baths, color healing, massage, and vitamin supplements were all part of the routine as well. He used laetrile, a substance derived from apricot or almond pits that is believed by some to be a cancer remedy. He applied acupuncture, a Chinese medical practice that attempts to cure illness by puncturing specified areas of the skin with needles. Gary also strongly believed in purifying the system twice a day through a high enema known as a colonic.

I don't know how you feel about colonics, but let me recount an experience that I'd had a few years earlier. As I was driving along Olympic Boulevard on a beautiful Saturday morning in Santa Monica just a few days before my thirty-fourth birthday, I suddenly had an overwhelming urge to buy myself a birthday present—a colonic. To this day, I still don't know where that desire came from. Maybe it was impending middle age, perhaps my family's colon cancer history also influenced me. I probably had just seen too many ads in the underground *L.A. Weekly* newspaper touting the procedure's remarkable benefits. According to the ads, which featured a misshapen, twisted colon, a colonic could cure depression, gas, fatigue, and even unemployment.

I imagined my middle-aged colon as a knotted, blackened cesspool of despair and destruction (the *Blade Runner* of bowels) and I figured I needed to clean that sucker right out. I thought I might even be able to rid my system of that bacon cheeseburger I'd had such a hard time digesting in 1961. Jim, the manager of a Venice health food store whose very clear skin suggested that he would have a lead on a colonic, directed me to a bulletin board where a prominently displayed COLONICS sign listed a phone number. I called and the next thing I knew, I was in somebody's living room wondering what the hell I had committed myself to. A little woman whose skin texture could best be described as raisinesque greeted me. She had beady brown eyes and wore a lavender shawl over her hair. She looked like a George Lucas creature, possibly Yoda's best friend.

She sidled over to me, smiled, and said, "You're next." Her voice had the quality of a gravel driveway. I think she immediately intuited my anxiety because she said, "Don't worry, you'll control the water pressure." Great, I thought. I got up and followed her into the room where I was to take off my clothes and put on a brown smock. I lay on the colonic table and felt like a Thanksgiving turkey on the big day. Standing over me was this little Ewok holding an ominous-looking nozzle in her very withered hands.

When she suddenly leaned over and said, "Are you ready?" I halfheartedly said, "Yes." "Tell me," she said. "What is Erik Estrada really like?" I sat there thinking, "You've got to be kidding me. I mean, is this God's joke? Is he laughing at me and teaching me a new meaning for the words *celebrity status* or what?"

Avoiding the question, I asked her to tell me about the glass tube on the machine. She explained it was the view tube. Now, I love television (especially cable), but the idea of watching what was coming out of my body seemed a little bizarre. But I went through with the procedure and interestingly enough, the only thing of any significance that I saw float by was one marijuana seed, probably from some brownies I had in 1969.

Ultimately, I don't think a colonic is natural. I think anyone who puts a hose up his ass has got to be a little strange. The truth is I had perfect intestinal health until that day. Took me years to recover. I think enemas and colemas are fine, but I just don't think machine-driven water is meant to be shot up your rectum.

Well, that was my total holistic experience. Yet there I was in a cancer clinic in Tijuana hugging my wife good-bye because this was the path she had chosen. I checked her into the clinic that afternoon for a three-week stay.

When Francesca returned home from Mexico three weeks later, she was radiant. Her eyes sparkled blue and her skin was silky smooth. She looked vibrant and alive.

Ready for a long fight, she cut her hair very short. She bought a T-shirt that had a picture of a shark on the front. Where the breast had been, the shark had a big open mouth looking as if it had just taken a huge bite. "Cancer humor," she said. Francesca would do anything to win this battle. Continuing Gary Young's program at home, she stuck to a vegetarian diet and squeezed fresh juices daily. She swallowed pills, vitamins, and supplements by the handful, took laetrile and practiced color healing, and continued home colonics. Every day she prayed to God and wrote in her journal. She said affirmations, did visualizations, and continued to read and network. She saw therapists, spiritualists, and psychics. All because she had cancer. She desperately wanted to get well. For herself, for me, for our children.

Francesca decided to supplement Gary's program by meeting with other healers. One afternoon a friend took her to a tent on the cliffs of Santa Monica, where she was granted a private audience with Muktananda, a visiting Indian guru. This beloved guru had her urinate into a glass jar. He stirred it with a peacock feather, read her urine, laughed, tickled her, tapped her on the forehead, and gave her a blessing before sending her on her way. Later that same friend told Francesca that Muktananda was very worried about her. Chex was both angered and frightened by her friend's negative, fear-provoking comments.

Francesca next called Louise Hay, the author of one of her favorite books, *Heal Yourself,* to make an appointment for a private session. They talked about the importance of getting in touch with the healing part of one's self.

Francesca's father put her in touch with Norman Cousins, now deceased. She spent two hours with him in his UCLA office talking about the importance of laughter and keeping one's chin up.

She contacted Dr. Bernie Siegel of *Love, Medicine and Miracles* fame. He asked her to draw pictures of her tumor and the cells attacking them. She mailed them to Dr. Siegel in Massachusetts.

He called and told her that she was too much of a "damn pacifist" and that she'd better draw those pictures again and really see herself as killing the cancer. Well, the phone call devastated her. She cried to me, "Paul, I guess I can't even kill my own cancer."

One afternoon, I walked into our kitchen to find her busy at the stove. The cutting board was out, and on it was a headless, tailless rattlesnake that our housekeeper, Josita, had arranged to have sent up from Guatemala. With a huge knife in her hand, Chex furiously chopped this reptile into little pieces, dropped them into the black skillet, and cooked them over a medium heat.

By the time she was done about three or four hours later, the rattlesnake was reduced to a saltlike powder that she sprinkled on her food for power. Enormously curious, I swiped some of the residue left in the pan with my finger to taste the "power" powder. Angrily, Chex scolded, "Don't you know how much that snake cost? Two hundred fifty dollars."

Chex fire walked on a twelve-foot bed of 2,200-degree coals because she believed that if she could overcome her fear of fire she would be empowered to conquer her disease. Fortunately, she didn't get a single burn and the experience was tremendously uplifting for her.

She saw a psychic surgeon, a sweet and funny little man named Oscar who was in California on a visit from the Philippines and practicing out of someone's home in West Covina. He smiled a lot at me and talked about how much he liked to play golf. Fascinated by the notion of taking a psychic surgeon onto the golf course, I wondered if he was a good putter and wanted to play eighteen holes with him.

When it was time for Oscar to begin, we were all summoned into the living room of the sprawling California ranch house. Almost fifty people gathered in front of a slightly elevated "operating" table, which created an altarlike appearance. I felt as if I was at a religious event as one by one, the "patients" went up and lay down on the massage table where the "surgeon" asked about their problem. He would then place his hands on the area of complaint while softly giving orders to his two female aides. To the naked eye, he appeared to be reaching inside each person's body; causing a bloodlike substance to appear. It didn't have the viscosity of real blood, but I thought of it as psychic blood. He then appeared to pull stringy, sinewy, tissuelike substances out of the body. I was ten feet away and didn't know what to believe. It looked real, but there was a close-up magic feel to it all.

Finally it was Francesca's turn. He asked everyone to turn away because her chest was going to be exposed. When I remained facing forward, the guy in front of me said, "You got to turn around, you got to turn around." I said, "It's okay, she's my wife, I've seen it."

Sure enough, Oscar "reached" into her chest and pulled out all this stuff. Once the gunk was extracted, he put it in a little silver pan, and it was taken away so fast that I never got a good chance to examine it.

I had him work on me just for the heck of it. When he asked what my difficulty was, I said, "I have abdominal problems." (Probably the result of that damn colonic.) He poked around and proclaimed me healthy.

It was an amazing "culture clash" evening. This man was not in it for the money. For him, this was purely a spiritual practice. The only monies exchanged were on a donation basis.

Chex had a number of sessions with Oscar. She always came away filled with hope, I doubt, however, that she was helped by them at all except psychically.

A month after Francesca's return from her initial visit to the Health and Life Clinic, I heard her scream from the bathroom and rushed upstairs to see what had happened. I found her naked from the waist up staring into the medicine cabinet mirror.

As I tried to get a sense of what was going on, she kept saying, "Look at this, look, look," pointing to the line of her incision, where there was a spot that looked like a tiny red blister. I thought it was just an irritation from the bandages that she was still wearing.

I tried to reassure her. "Chex, it's just a little blister."

"No, no, it's not," she said adamantly. "I know it's not. It's back. Goddamnit. Why? Why me? It's back, Paul, it's back."

She called the Health and Life Clinic immediately and was on her way back down south of the border the next day. I didn't go with her this time. Gary gave her a "pulling salve," a brownish ointment that he told her to apply to her wound.

She began the process of pulling the tumor out of her chest. It was a long, very painful procedure. The salve literally drew the tumor to the surface, where it formed a quarter-sized, callous scab. After a while, it began to separate from her chest, which created ooze and blood. Slowly but surely, the scab flaked off.

Francesca was elated when it finally came off. When I didn't jump for joy, she became very angry with me.

"You don't care. You're not interested in what I'm doing. You don't understand the battle I'm in. How can you not understand and appreciate what I've just done?"

She led me upstairs to show me the tumor, which was now floating in a little jar of alcohol. It looked like a huge scab. I didn't consider it a big deal and my indifference offended her.

"You're not supporting me at all on this. You're totally in denial. You know I have cancer, I'm fighting for my life and I can't do this by myself. You don't give me any strokes. What's with you, Paul?"

"Of course, I'm happy for you," I lied. Actually, I was embarrassed by my own lack of interest and understanding. I retreated into my shell, remaining stuck in my denial.

The tumor that fell off had left a small hole. From it another tumor, which was a little bit bigger, began to form. Once she pulled that one out, a slightly larger hole was left and yet another tumor appeared. Ultimately, she pulled three or four tumors out of her chest. The last one was the size of a silver dollar.

Her cancer was now visible, and additional tumors had sprung up along the scar line from her sternum to the underarm area. Francesca blamed the operation for the rapid growth of the malignancy, which she felt was fueled by the direct exposure to air. Ironically, to her dying day, the only remedy she regretted was the mastectomy.

Angered by the three traditional medical options—cut, burn or poison—Francesca felt isolated in her holistic beliefs. She had become the lone Warrior Woman.

The Chart House

"What do you think I should do?"
"All you ever talk about anymore is ...cancer."

I walked into our bedroom one afternoon and found Chex in the midst of her daily wellness program. Sitting under the color lamp, she held a crystal while listening to a self-help tape. I suggested that we write a book about her adventures in alternative healing.

"You know, we've got to write a book about this. People don't understand. When someone is diagnosed with cancer, they are forced into a world of terrifying choices, particularly if they take an alternative path. Watching you, I've discovered how complicated, how involved, how strange, how different it all is. I think people would be fascinated by what it means to do what you're doing. I can see it now, *My Wife Has Cancer. A Handbook of Alternative Cancer Therapies.*"

She immediately fired back, "No, no. *My Wife Had Cancer.*"

I looked at her and said, "I'll tell you what. Let's call it *My Wife Has Cancer* and we'll attach a pencil with a string to the binding of each book. If you've won your battle, we'll let them cross out 'has' and write 'had.'"

She wasn't amused. I made jokes to lighten her up, but she found very little funny. We had lost a crucial component of our relationship—laughter.

Mealtime was especially difficult for us. While the boys and I would enjoy our favorite foods, she would pick at her

67

unappetizing vegetarian fare. Chex was quick to comment on the toxicity of everything we liked to eat.

Sex stopped altogether. Chex was exhausted and so put off by my self-absorption that she did not feel close enough to me for intimacy. And because of her endless fatigue, she could no longer keep up with our two young boys. She was just too drained to be a wife and mother. Cancer was her life, and our home had turned into the battlefield on which this grim war was waged.

I decided we needed a night out together—a date—to take a break from the madness and try to rekindle our ebbing love affair.

We went to our favorite restaurant, The Chart House in Marina Del Rey. As we stood at the salad bar, I had dug deeply for two ice cold plates when Chex brought up the one topic that I didn't want to discuss. She had seen a man on "Donahue" that day who had beaten cancer through a whole new approach. I silently began to burn as we created our salads. This was not how "our night" was supposed to be, so I ignored her comments.

But at our table, Chex continued to press me.

"What do you think, Paul? Does this sound like a way for me to go? Should I leave Gary's program?"

In the soft candlelight, I suddenly lost my appetite for it *all*. I looked down at my uneaten food and took a deep breath as she continued.

"Maybe I should contact Donahue...they could put me in touch with this man. Maybe it was a sign from God. Tell me... what do you think I should do? Talk to me, Paul."

I lost control. "Goddamnit, Francesca! FUCK! JESUS CHRIST! All you ever talk about anymore is fucking CANCER. I've had it up to HERE with this shit! Look at me, Francesca. Goddamnit. LOOK AT ME! I'M ALIVE. RIGHT HERE, RIGHT NOW. My heart is beating in my chest and the blood is running through my veins, but you don't see me anymore. You don't see our kids anymore. All you care about is your fucking disease! Goddamnit."

The ferocity of my outburst stunned us both into silence. Almost on cue, our waiter appeared with a basket of rolls. We picked at our plates and carefully avoided each other's glances. It was not until our entrées arrived that I saw the glistening tears on her cheeks. It was the moment in which my denial was expunged by the rage hidden beneath. I could no longer evade the dominant issue in our lives. I needed to be compassionate and show understanding in order to grow as husband, father, and man.

Cancer is hard. It affects the whole family. We ate the rest of our dinner in silence, and the guilt I felt after the explosion lasted for years.

The Miracle of Rose

"Papa, I love you so much. I love you past Pluto."

A couple of months after her return from the clinic, Francesca's healthy glow had faded and she felt terrible all the time. Daily nausea made her fear she might be pregnant. Frantic, she went to the L.A. Childbirth Center and had a pregnancy test. When the results came back negative, she assumed the symptoms were part of her "healing crisis" and continued her program.

One month later, when her condition hadn't improved, she had a second pregnancy test done just in case. Again, the results were negative. Convinced she was dying after four months of feeling poorly, Chex rushed back to Tijuana with hope that Gary would help her get well again.

Chex called me from the clinic a few days later. She wanted to see me so we could talk. We decided to meet in La Jolla. My mother lived there and the boys could visit with her while Chex and I spent time together.

The boys and I arrived in La Jolla and checked into room 23 at the Inn at La Jolla. I wasn't sure when Chex was going to show up, so I took the hungry guys out for pizza. Francesca joined us later at the restaurant, but there was nothing for her to eat on the menu. Things were tense while the boys finished up their dinner, but I figured she was just tired. We went back to the motel and put the kids to bed. After Chex made some of her special herbal tea, she joined me in the living room of our little suite to talk.

She put her cup down on the coffee table, sat in a chair opposite me, and said, "Paul, Gary doesn't understand why I'm not getting well and I don't understand why I'm not getting well either. His program works. I haven't cheated one time. But let's face it. It isn't working for me. I am not getting better. Those kids in there need a mom. Last night, Gary and I talked about my relationship with you. Gary thinks that maybe my problem is you."

"What?" I muttered in disbelief.

"He thinks that maybe your anger is in the way of my getting well. I need positive energy around me to beat this thing. So this is what I want to do, Paul. When I come home from the clinic next week, I want you to move out of the house. I want you to find another place to live. I'm sorry, but I have to do this. I need space from you. I need to concentrate on getting well and I can't do it with you in our home."

Her message crashed over me like a huge wave that had slowly formed out at sea before breaking on the shore. Hurt and angry, I felt like a drowning man struggling for air in a desperate attempt to survive. My wife, the mother of my two children, had cancer, had a mastectomy, and now she wanted me to leave.

"Okay," I said through clenched teeth. "If that's what you want."

The boys and I returned home the next morning. I had agreed to move out when Francesca returned. Five days later while sitting at our dining-room table, I gazed out into the backyard, where all the neighborhood kids played. They were running pell-mell around the plum tree enjoying their little lives. My eyes drifted over to the orange tree, where one blossom caught my attention. I mused about the odd course that my life had suddenly taken. The phone rang and broke my contemplation. It was Francesca calling me again from Tijuana.

"I'm sorry, Paul, I am so sorry. I don't know what I was thinking. I don't want you to leave me. I need you in my life now more than ever. I'm just so scared. I just want to get well, Goddamnit. Can you forgive me? Please, sweetheart. I guess I'm just your freaked-out girl. Forgive me. Guess what, Paul, I found something out today. Are you sitting down? This is going to blow your mind. I am pregnant."

The room revolved rapidly like a vomit-inducing, antigravity amusement park ride. As the freshly brewed "news" filtered through the Melitta of my mind, I reassessed my situation: I've got a wife and two kids. She has cancer and had a mastectomy. She wanted me to leave, now she wants me to stay. And we're going to welcome a newborn into the middle of *this* chaos?

A week later, Francesca was back at home. One afternoon I found her on the phone engaged in a heated conversation with her surgeon, Dr. Karlin. She looked at me in exasperation. "Yes, I heard what you said, Dr. Karlin. But the problem is you never hear what I'm saying. See, there you go again. You have got to learn to listen to me. Look, Dr. Karlin, I'm having this baby. Yes, I understand, but I'm telling you that I am going to deliver this baby at term. One day, Dr. Karlin, I will walk into your office with a beautiful healthy baby as a cancer survivor, all right? Thank you, thank you very much, Dr. Karlin. Now good-bye."

Agitated, she said, "Can you believe that man, Paul? Calling me up at my home to see if I'm still working with that clinic and when he finds out I'm pregnant, he goes absolutely nuts. He screamed at me. Do you know what he wants me to do, Paul? He wants me to have an abortion. Think about it. I'm four and a half months pregnant, I have cancer. Would you tell me how my body's supposed to survive an abortion? I am fighting to save my own life and he wants me to end the life inside me. How can that be life-affirming? How can that be the right thing for me to do, Paul? Tell me."

Now what she *didn't* tell me that day, and didn't share with me until she was dying, were Dr. Karlin's exact words. What he said that so upset her was that if she went ahead and delivered the baby at term, she would be dead within one year of the birth of the child. Ultimately, she lived one year and three days after our third child's birth.

The worst possible scenario for a female cancer patient is pregnancy. A woman's body goes into a state of temporary remission that is totally illusory. What's really going on is that her body is giving all its strength and energy to that cocooning fetus inside. After the baby is born, the postpartum hormone balance shifts and sets itself up to blaze like a wildfire. Kind of like the bone-dry hills of southern California in Santa Ana conditions. They're just ripe for some asshole motorist with zero consciousness who flicks his still-burning cigarette out of his car window into the roadside brush.

Just as that hillside would explode into flames, so would Francesca's life force be consumed after the birth of our third baby.

This unexpected pregnancy was also a surprise to the L.A. Childbirth Center. The doctor affiliated with the birth center did extensive research before concluding that the pregnancy and birth would be no problem and gave the go-ahead for a third home birth. He felt that the baby would be fine, but Francesca would be in danger after the birth. He advised her to nurse the baby for a very short time.

March 24, 1985. "Vi!" Francesca screamed, "I feel like I'm going to die. I can't handle it."

"You're doing great, Francesca," Vi said. "You're doing beautifully.

"I've got to change positions," she said. "I want to squat."

Vi and I helped her off the water bed so she could squat. Chex immediately began to push. The hood was up, so to speak, and Vi, our Mr. Goodwrench, worked under her. I wanted to catch my third child just as I had caught Ryan, but I was too busy rubbing Francesca's back and neck to grasp our new arrival. At 3:00 A.M., our little daughter, Rose, was born, my blond-haired girl who now says things to me like, "Papa, I love you so much. I love you past Pluto."

There was one conversation that Francesca and I had over and over again when she was dying. "You know something, Paul. All this time, through this whole cancer thing, I always prayed to God for a miracle. I always thought that the miracle that I was praying for was to get well, to be healed. I know now that I'm getting my healing, but my healing is going to happen outside of my body. And we got our miracle, Paul. The miracle is Rose."

Grains and Greens

"Gary, I'm pregnant..."
"...I want you to fast for a month."

There is a lot of irony in the fact that Francesca found out she was pregnant while at the clinic in Tijuana and that both tests taken in the United States were negative. Perhaps if she had learned about her pregnancy earlier, she might have considered an abortion. Who knows?

Chex went into Gary's office to tell him the news from the lab. Gary was thrilled for her, and his first suggestion was that she begin a thirty-to-forty day fast of juice and water.

That was the moment that Francesca decided to leave Gary's program. She refused to punish her body or the fetus inside her by undergoing such a strict and stringent program. She came back home without any ideas about the next step in her ongoing treatment.

At the suggestion of her brother, Willy, she began working with Dr. John, a chiropractor from Boulder who had studied with a famous healer in Oregon. He used an eclectic approach. It involved rather large, foul-tasting pills that she had to chew. He performed acupuncture, therapeutic massage, and a lot of muscle testing for food allergies. He put her on a very strict diet of pressure-cooked grains and steamed vegetables. Every twenty-first meal, she was permitted a few ounces of fish for protein. This meager diet was a real struggle for Chex, but she did it.

Once a month, Dr. John flew to Los Angeles, at our expense, to spend the weekend with us. He stayed in our home, ate our food (he didn't use much salad dressing), used our car, and charged us one hundred dollars an hour. These weekends averaged over a thousand dollars, plus airfare.

My insurance didn't cover these treatments, so her father pitched in and paid for them. While under Dr. John's care, she looked great. She was lean, mean, and vital. You never would have guessed that she was ill with a life-threatening disease.

I was still in my unconscious mode, overweight and continuing to eat steak. I couldn't understand why Dr. John was so uptight about a little oil in salad dressing. Dr. John took Francesca all the way through her pregnancy. She felt good working with him and rigidly adhered to his precepts. She bought a special Iranian pressure cooker to prepare grains and used gomazio, a special seasoning of sesame seed and salt. She was a real trooper and once again, she was filled with hope. I too was hopeful that she would conquer her cancer.

The Breast Center

"I'd cut everything from here... to here."

Shortly after Rose was born, Francesca decided to seek conventional medical help. Seeing her beautiful baby girl fueled her desire to conquer cancer with whatever means it took. Our friend Deirdre had had a biopsy performed on a suspicious lump at a woman's clinic. Deirdre's positive experience at the center spurred Chex to have the people there check her out.

We arrived at the medical building on a very hot afternoon with two-month-old Rose. We were both in a positive frame of mind as we sat in the calm yet bustling waiting room. I felt the environment was conducive to helping women and was grateful to Francesca for taking the step.

After a short wait, the three of us were ushered into an examination room where we waited for the doctor to join us. The sliding door opened and in walked an older male doctor who was a cross between Abe Lincoln and Morton Downey, Jr.

After listening to Francesca's case history, the doctor directed her to remove her blouse and bandage for an exam. He appeared to be taken aback by the sight of her external tumors. He was pensive for a few moments before offering his opinion. He removed a red pen from his lab coat pocket and drew red dots around the infected area. He then proceeded to connect the dots, thereby creating a pie-shaped diagram on her skin. He then gave us his preferred plan of attack, which was to surgically remove the entire wedge. To me, it resembled a hunk of Jarlsberg cheese cut from the wheel.

"I'd cut everything from here to here," he stated.

Chex was aghast. She was grossly offended at being treated like a sketch pad and was incredulous at his suggestion.

"If you cut from here to here," she asked, "how do you close the gap?"

"Oh, don't worry about that," he said, unilaterally dismissing her fears. "That won't be a problem."

He excused himself and left us there to ponder our predicament. "That guy's out of his mind," Chex commented.

While we sat there, the sliding door opened again. A nurse looked in for a moment before she said, "Oh, excuse me, I must have the wrong room," and shut the door. Another minute passed by and the same thing happened again. Only this time there were two nurses who gaped at Chex's exposed cancer before excusing themselves. After the third such incident, we knew that we were the main attraction in a medical freak show. We were left with the distinct impression that none of the peeping medical personnel had ever seen cancer up close before. We also suspected that the staff had been briefed and directed to "check out room A." Our doctor never showed his face again.

The continuous opening-closing of the sliding door woke a sleeping Rose, who promptly started to scream her head off.

There we were, a supine Chex, a bawling Rose, and a helpless Paul. We were trapped in the hot, tiny room and desperate to escape.

Finally, a different doctor appeared. He was a young, kind, and gentle man with an entirely different attitude. He bandaged Chex back up and held Rose while she dressed. He said that he didn't think surgery was a viable option. He was very forthright and talked about chemotherapy. While he wished he could

80

help, in his opinion it was too late for chemo to be effective.

This was her last attempt to reach out to the conventional medical world for its help. When most of us have a pain, we fear the worst and seek medical advice. Usually, it turns out to be nothing, and we are treated and sent off on our way. In Francesca's case, however, every time she walked into those offices, it turned out to be the worst-case scenario.

As we drove home, our conversation focused on the insensitivity of her treatment at this supposedly female-oriented clinic. What we were unable to bring out into the open was the prognosis. It was still too early for us to understand that it was too late.

Sex and the Single Sikh

"Marriage is the ultimate dance...the gateway to infinity."

During Francesca's pregnancy and postpartum, anger permeated the fabric of our relationship. Chex felt that I didn't give her the support she needed and that I was an angry man. I felt I had no life and resented the absence of sexuality in our marriage. The children had their needs and Francesca had her needs. What about me? I'm a very physical person and desperately missed having sex.

My male friends and I discussed our marital dilemmas and discovered a common grievance. It seemed that after our wives had children, sex ended. I came up with a theory that the milk that our wives produced for our children was drawn from the cream that used to emanate from between their legs. They all laughed, but I think they agreed with me. I now recognize it as an aspect of life and marriage. But my situation was compounded by cancer.

Under the best circumstances, marriage is a tremendous test. When you add in the elements of little children and a life-threatening disease, the daily trials become even more challenging.

I had a lot on my plate, so I began to see a therapist to help me navigate these treacherous marital waters. Satkaur Khalsa was a practicing Sikh who wore white robes and a turban. She was a follower of Yogi Baghwan.

Satkaur told me that marriage was the gateway to infinity and the ultimate dance we do. If that was true, then Francesca and I were stumbling over each other's feet of fear and anger. We were in the pit and sinking.

During one session, Satkaur talked about the courtship ritual within marriage from a spiritual perspective. It was her notion that in the course of each month, there were a few days of intense courting finally consummated by sexual intercourse. The bottom line was—sex once a month.

The irony of it all made me laugh. I had sought therapy to deal with my anger at not getting laid and wound up being counseled by a woman who believed in having sex once a month. I figured it must be God's sense of humor at work.

Looking back, I recognize that my therapy was a turning point in our relationship. In an effort to achieve greater understanding about my wife and myself, I had unknowingly begun the process of reconciliation.

Getting Our Salad Together
and Taking It on the Road

*"Chex, go out on the lake ... You need those positive
ions around you."*

T he summer of 1985 was the Linkes' last family vacation. We
spent it with two dozen close friends at the Appleton Lodge
in the north woods of Wisconsin. It was two weeks of fun in the
sun and lake play too. It was a major undertaking for our family,
traveling with two spirited little boys, a newborn child, and a sick
wife on a "grains and greens diet." We transported almost eighty
pounds of food with us so that Chex could stay on her program.
It wouldn't be easy, but we wanted to have this time together.

About two weeks before we left, I experienced a moment of
spiritual reawakening. This unexpected milestone took place
when I accompanied Francesca out to Topanga Canyon, an
enclave of diverse lifestyles tucked into the Santa Monica mountains. We had been invited to a potluck celebration to honor
Chex's therapist, Dina Metzger.

Dina, a small, gypsy-type bohemian woman, was a fairly well-
known local poet. She was giving up her therapy practice to
concentrate on writing. Having survived cancer herself, she was
an important ally to Francesca. She had lived to talk about her
own mastectomy sixteen years earlier and had helped many
women through theirs. Francesca once told me that Dina had a
tattoo of a clinging vine etched on her chest where her breast

had been. She felt that the tattoo gave people permission to look at her chest which was especially important in southern California, where getting in a hot tub with a few people was a critical aspect of life.

I was a reluctant escort/guest at the dinner and had only gone along to demonstrate my support to Francesca. I dutifully carried our covered-dish offering of turkey curry up the steep hill to Dina's house, where an eclectic group of people had gathered around an incredible array of food. I scarfed some of the curry and sampled other goodies while Chex made the rounds and talked to people. Just as the sun set, an actor friend, Linden Childes, walked into the garden where I was enjoying the last bit of daylight. I was on the defensive because I had not cast him in a play that I had directed five months earlier.

I finally got up the nerve to ask him how he was doing.

"Not very well," was his reply. He paused before saying, "I'm having a really hard time. My twenty-three-year-old son was killed in a car accident a couple of weeks ago on the Pacific Coast Highway... it's really rough right now."

I was absolutely stunned and didn't know what to say. Linden recalled how he had actually driven by the scene of the accident and sensed that someone had died, but he had no idea that it was his own son.

We talked for hours. Being a parent, I dread the thought of ever losing a child and couldn't get over how well he was coping with his loss. I was in awe of his spirituality and overwhelming sense of serenity. I don't remember specifically what he said, but somewhere in the middle of the conversation it became totally clear to me (a fervent ex-Catholic) that I had the right to choose to believe in a higher power.

I had not considered the spiritual aspects of life for a long time. As far as Catholicism goes, I didn't buy the ideas pumped into my brain way back then at St. Dominic's in Oyster Bay, Long Island. I could never accept confession. As a six- or seven-year-old boy, I went into the confessional and had to search for sins. What could a seven-year-old boy possibly have to confess? By the age of eight, I had decided that the Church was not for me. A brief flirtation occurred again in my teenage years, when my father prepared to convert to Catholicism in order to join my mother's faith. It ended one boring Sunday morning in church when I randomly opened his catechism. There in bold italics were those fateful words: MASTURBATION IS A MORTAL SIN. I closed the book and terminated my Catholic career.

Listening to Linden talk about the loss of his son triggered a spiritual renewal in me. After many years of indifference to God, I realized that there had to be more going on than we could see and we were truly all a part of God's tapestry. It's simply a binary concept, A or B. Positive or negative. It comes down to choice: whichever one you make, that is the perspective from which you will live your life, the point of view through which you will see the world.

A few days after Dina's bash, I was in the bookstore getting the kids some goodies for the dreaded plane ride to the lodge. Paying at the cash register, I noticed a stack of books in the front of the store. On top was *Goodbye to Guilt* by Jerry Jampolsky. Something told me I needed to read that book immediately.

After a long day on airplanes, we finally arrived at the Appleton Lodge, a beautiful old hunting retreat that sits on an isthmus between Harmony Lake and Butternut Lake. We were there with old college friends and their children to recreate by day and party by night.

One of the things about the Appleton Lodge is its intention to fill you up with hearty American food—bacon-and-egg breakfasts with sweet rolls, cold-cut lunches, barbecued-steak-and-baked-potato dinners, heavy desserts, and snacks. It served very few fruits and vegetables. To a Wisconsinite, if you don't have meat, it's not a meal.

On our arrival, we went straight to Julie, the cook, to explain Francesca's situation. Julie and her staff were a little dumbfounded by the stacks of boxes that had suddenly invaded their well-ordered kitchen. We hastily explained that we didn't want to cause any trouble, but Chex was ill and required a special diet. We were given our own cooking area downstairs and away from the flow of the main kitchen, which was responsible for cranking out three meals a day for twenty-four people.

Every evening after dinner, my dear friend Albert would pilot the lodge's pontoon boat, *African Queen*, onto Butternut Lake, with all his guests aboard, to celebrate the sunset.

On the fifth night, as we all prepared to board the *Queen* for the "sunset special," Francesca told me she was too tired to come and would rather stay behind. I tried to persuade her to come since it was always one of the highlights of the trip. I offered to stay behind and babysit Rose and finally convinced her to go by saying, "Chex, go out on the lake. You need those positive ions around you."

I sat in a lawn chair on the hillside overlooking the lake below. With Rose asleep on a blanket at my feet, I settled in to read my new book, *Goodbye to Guilt*.

About thirty minutes later, the pontoon boat approached the dock to unload its passengers. As it got closer, I looked out at all the faces of my lake-faring friends. They were all so happy and celebrating the summer of their lives. The kids were running around the boat; one honeymooning couple necked at the stern. Everyone was so vital and alive. My eyes found a pallid Francesca, who quietly sat on the far side of the boat on a long padded bench under the blue-striped awning. She appeared to be lost in deep thought, oblivious to all the teeming life that swirled around her. My vantage point gave me a new perspective. Everyone on that pontoon boat had a hundred-watt bulb in their sockets except for my fragile Francesca, who had a ten-watt bulb in hers. It was dimming and flickering in front of my eyes. Time stood still. I knew she was dying.

I wanted to take this realization and hurl it into the sky like Thor's thunderbolt. Instead, I put it on hold by picking up my copy of *Goodbye to Guilt* and settling back for the rest of our two-week family vacation.

The Rest of 1985

"Paul, why are you here?...
"I want to heal my relationship."

I finished *Goodbye to Guilt* in Wisconsin and was so impressed with what Jerry Jampolsky had to say, I decided I wanted to meet him. The Attitudinal Healing Center in Tiburon, California, informed me about a workshop that was being held the last weekend in August. It was called a Facilitator's Training Conference. Jerry was scheduled to open the conference and there was still space available.

I had no idea what a Facilitator's Training Conference was, but I wanted to meet Jerry, so I made arrangements to attend the weekend. The very next day, I talked to my friend Julie, who lived in San Francisco, and told her I was coming up to meet Jerry. Not only did I learn that they were friends, but she offered to send him a personal note of introduction on my behalf.

I spent the fourth weekend of August 1985 at Dominican College in San Rafael, California. Right before the conference was scheduled to begin, I sat out in the open courtyard, hoping to catch a glimpse of Jerry before the start of the program. As soon as I saw him enter, I approached him and introduced myself.

"Hi, Jerry. My name is Paul Linke."

He smiled and with a twinkle in his eye said, "I was looking for you. Sit down." We sat down and he asked, "Paul, why are you here?"

"Jerry, I read your book, *Goodbye to Guilt*. It is so fantastic. You are able to talk about what's going on inside us."

"Paul," he repeated, "why are you here?"

There was a long pause while I came to terms with the true meaning of his question.

"I think my wife is dying of cancer, Jerry. I want to heal my relationship with her."

Perhaps life is really this simple. Maybe when it comes right down to it, it's simply a matter of stating our wishes out loud, claiming them as ours, visualizing them, and then actively making a choice.

Three days later, I returned from the conference, walked into the kitchen, and hugged Francesca. She pulled back to look at me.

"My God, what happened to you up there? You've changed."

Our healing had begun.

The rest of 1985 went by like one of those old movies where the calendar pages miraculously rip themselves off the wall and gently float down into the cylindrical trash can below.

By this point, I was responsible for all the driving, all the shopping, and all the cooking. I invented "nouvelle kiddeaux," a low-fat anticancer diet for the tiny tots that featured the many forms of hormone-less turkey. Proteins and carbohydrates were never mixed. Each and every dinner had an array of al dente garden vegetables fanned beautifully around the edges of their plates. The kids were absolutely horrified by this food.

"Kids, if you clean your plates, you'll get a great dessert that has no sugar and no honey," I would joke.

Francesca had lost faith and interest in continuing her treatment with Dr. John. Those weekend visits had taken their toll financially, emotionally, and physically. She felt she'd gone as far as she could with him. In a slight panic, she tried to figure out her next move.

One November morning, I found Francesca standing in the bathroom nude. The Draper ass was gone. She'd had a great ass.

That afternoon I saw that her back was one long straight line. She had lost weight right in front of my eyes and was fading away. Shocked by this sudden realization, I yelled at her, "Goddamnit, Francesca, this fucking grains and greens diet is not working. Honey, isn't there something else we could do for you? Is there some other approach you'd like to try? Anything?"

With a sad smile, she said, "I've always wanted to go to the Hoxsey Clinic, Paul."

"Okay," I said. "I'll call them up and make all the arrangements for you." We hugged and proceeded to go about the business of what was to become the Linkes' last family Christmas.

We decorated the tree. Francesca stood at the mantel over the fireplace and arranged the figures of our little créche. I finished stringing the lights and turned the whole operation over to Jasper, our artist-in-residence, to work his magic. I watched him cover the tree with the ornaments that Chex and I had accumulated during our marriage. Rosie sat with me on the couch while Ryan played on the floor. The scene overwhelmed me and I began to cry. I knew it was going to be the last Christmas the five of us would spend together.

But I didn't want to spoil the evening for everyone, so I dried my eyes and went about the business at hand in denial.

I wanted to make it an extra-special Christmas for Chex. I gave her diamond stud earrings because I wanted her to be hard. I wanted to give her a cobalt-blue leather dress to make her tough. I saw the color clearly in my mind and scoured L.A. for the dress. The only store that had it wanted $2,500 for it. Depressed, I gave up. I finally found something close to what I had in mind at a trendy Westside mall. While I was taking a breather from Christmas shopping, I spotted a red chamois dress in the front window of a chic boutique. As soon as I saw that it had snakeskin on it, I bought it.

I had hoped that these accoutrements would inspire Francesca. I believed that my Warrior Woman needed to be hard as diamonds and tough as leather to face the ultimate battle before her in 1986.

Hoxsey Clinic

"How much do you want her to know?... It's bad, it's really bad."

J anuary 6, 1986. I'd made arrangements to take Chex to the Hoxsey Clinic, a treatment center in Tijuana that claimed to have an herbal cure for cancer. And so one more time, we were leaving the country in search of a miracle. The doorway to the Hoxsey is through the International Motel, which sits on the United States-Mexico border just below San Ysidro. This funky little motel serves as a conduit to the outpatient Hoxsey Biomedico, which is south of the border.

After a horrible night's sleep, we stood in front of the office at 8:00 a.m. to await the van from the clinic. It pulled into the courtyard and the peppy driver, J. Raul Coria, rolled down his window and yelled, "Hoxsey Biomedico."

At least forty people from all over the world suddenly started to stream out of various motel rooms (like rats from a sinking ship). All had come to seek their healing. It took three van loads and practically two and a half hours before we were all shuttled south of the border. I let Chex go ahead with other patients while I waited and took the last van. I talked to Raul about the Hoxsey as we crossed the border. He explained the history of the clinic. It was a hillside mansion built by one of Tijuana's major drug dealers for his wife-to-be, an infamous prostitute. Quite a couple, I thought. They both had been busted by the Federales, leaving their palace vacant. Mildred Nelson, director of the Hoxsey, had persuaded the city of Tijuana to allow her to use it for a clinic.

We drove up a hill through huge iron gates. A cobblestone driveway led up to the mansion. There was a large open-air aviary with exotic birds in the front. I went to find Francesca. As fate would have it, we had selected the busiest day of the year for the Hoxsey. It was their first open day after the holidays.

There were so many patients and the clinic was so short-staffed that it was hours before the staff saw Francesca. There were blood tests, X-rays, physical exams, and lots of time spent waiting. After lunch, we joined a group of new patients in a doctor's office, where we were to be taught how to mix the Hoxsey tonic, an herbal cure for cancer.

Francesca had always been fascinated by Harry Hoxsey. He had claimed to have found his cure many years before. It was based on research that he had begun after observing sick animals on his farm and their tendency to gravitate to a section of his property where particular weeds and herbs grew. They ate them and would get better. He concocted a formula based on those herbs.

At one point, Harry Hoxsey had cancer clinics all over the United States. But he and the American Medical Association did not see eye to eye. Specifically, he battled with the editor of the AMA journal. Ultimately, Hoxsey was driven out of the country and forced to practice in Mexico. From Francesca's research, we learned that the AMA had originally offered Hoxsey money for his formula. But in return, it had wanted total ownership. He balked at the terms and the rift began. Harry Hoxsey died in 1974, and the clinic was then placed in the hands of Mildred Nelson, who had originally gone there with her ailing mother. Mildred, a registered nurse, had arrived an absolute skeptic, but found that Hoxsey really helped people. She wound up staying and running the clinic.

While sitting in the doctor's office waiting to be taught the secrets of the Hoxsey tonic, I looked around the room. There were five other couples in the room that day. I looked at all these men and women dealing with catastrophic illnesses and thought to myself how fantastic it was that their mates were supporting them during these difficult times. I marveled at what I perceived as a reflection of love. I was brought back to earth by Dr. Fernando Ariola, who tapped me on the shoulder and asked me to follow him.

He led me through the corridor and into the director's office, where I finally met Mildred Nelson. She was talking on the telephone to someone in Europe about cancer. What a sight. Mildred was a petite, wiry woman in her late sixties who appeared to have lived in the desert most of her life and was sharp as a tack. Her dried, weathered skin was probably due to the brown Sherman cigarettes that she chain-smoked. Her crow's feet would qualify as wraparound sunglasses. She wore her graying blond hair pulled straight back in a ponytail and was super-intense with a double-expresso delivery. When she finally hung up about ten minutes later, Mildred removed her wire-rimmed glasses and greeted me with her steely blue eyes. "How much do you want her to know?"

"What?" I said.

"How much do you want her to know?" she continued. "Is she tough? Can she take it? It's bad. It's really bad."

"But Mildred," I said, "I don't know what you're talking about. Whatever there is for Francesca to know, she's got to know. This is her body we're talking about."

She slapped her hand on the desk and said, "Fine. I just wanted to check with you first. Now come with me, please."

She led me back up the same corridor and into a room with an X-ray unit on the wall. There were two separate sets of X rays clipped onto the unlit panels. She went to the first set, clicked on the lights, and said, "You see this chest X ray here? You see how these lungs are all black? These are healthy lungs."

She showed me the second set by clicking the light on. "Now, see this chest X ray here? See how these lungs are all white? Can you see that difference there? See how it's totally white? Well, they call that snowballing. That's all cancer. Those are your wife's lungs."

And in the moment that denial died for me forever, Francesca passed the open door. I called for her to join us. "Hey, Chex. You'd better look at this." Francesca instinctively knew what it meant. We silently embraced as Mildred clicked off the X ray panels.

We drove home in silence. It wasn't the same kind of silence we had on our first ride down to Mexico, one that was bound up in anger and fear. This silence expressed our confirmation and acceptance. Grief doesn't begin when somebody dies.

It's Hospice Time Again.
You're Going to Leave Me.

"You're not going to any hospital...I want you here ...
where you belong."

We returned home from the Hoxsey Clinic to mount our final assault. I was now an active participant in Francesca's struggle. I mixed her tonic, read her books, and networked with doctors and healers all around the country. I became her ally.

One week later, while preparing to head down to Venice Beach to play paddle tennis, my all-time favorite pastime, I went upstairs in search of a sturdy pair of Thor-lo socks. Chex was sitting on the edge of the water bed looking particularly fragile and pale. Words started to pour from my mouth that I didn't even know were in my heart.

"Chex, I want you to know something. No matter how sick you get, I'll take care of you. I'll be your nurse. You're not going to any hospital. I want you here with me and the kids where you belong. I'm in this with you all the way."

She looked at me and rivers of tears flowed from her eyes. I didn't know anything about hospices, but I wanted to do this for Chex.

In mid-January 1986, I went to see the Reverend Jim Conn, minister of the Church at Ocean Park. He had stood on the beach at Paradise Cove eight years earlier and under the rippling wedding flag had pronounced us husband and wife. We embraced, and he wept over the pain in our life. We talked for a while, and he made some suggestions to help Francesca and me on our journey.

First he gave me a copy of Stephen Levine's book *Who Dies: An Investigative Journal into Conscious Living and Conscious Dying*. He also gave me the name of Leni Wildflower, a woman who had lost her husband, Paul Potter, to pancreatic cancer a year and a half earlier at home in Santa Fe, New Mexico.

I called Leni and she agreed to meet me at the Rose Café. We sat and talked for a long time. I could tell she was still coming to terms with her own loss. She was sweet, funny, neurotic, and open. Uncertain as to how she could be of service to us, she thought that perhaps by sharing her experience with us, she might further her own healing. By helping us negotiate each stage of the dying process, she hoped to come full circle in coping with her loss.

Her husband died with Stephen Levine at his bedside. Leni laughed when she recalled his final hours. It seemed that while Stephen prayed for a peaceful crossing, her husband was annoyed that he was missing the Lakers-Celtics playoff game on television. We die the way we live.

Leni and Chex connected instantly and had a tearful first meeting in our bedroom. Leni provided support, information, and help whenever we needed it. She became our midwife in death and was truly an understanding guide because she had traveled the route.

Nothing remained for Francesca and me to do except take the Carlos Castaneda leap of faith. The bullshit was over and the game was up. We had turned to the final chapter of our loving and living together. We could no longer hide from it. We needed to open our hearts to the precious time that was left and use it to create something for ourselves, each other, and our kids. This conscious choice in approaching her death changed our perceptions and turned the darkest period of our lives into the best of times for Francesca and me.

100

Grand Central Station

"This is not about how I cut my yellow bell pepper...This is about your daughter, my wife, who is dying."

By the middle of February, Francesca's condition had deteriorated and she was bedridden. Her external tumors had grown quite large and her skin was rotting and smelled foul. She could no longer pick up the baby because the strain irritated the tumors.

One morning she woke up with a severe pain in her side. We called Mildred at the clinic, who suggested that Chex might have pleurisy, an inflammation of the lining of the lung. Mildred's suggestion that she try a sling to relieve some of the pressure helped a bit.

Francesca's mom, Bee, was due for her annual visit. Every year she left her Long Island home and came to southern California to escape the long, cold New York winter.

Bee was stunned by Chex's appearance. Shock registered in her eyes at first sight of her eldest daughter. They hadn't seen each other in a while and even though Bee knew Chex was struggling with cancer, she wasn't prepared for the condition in which she found her.

When you live with it day in, day out, the shift is gradual. Now when I look at photos of Francesca taken three weeks before her death, I am shocked by her physical appearance. Funny, I remember thinking at the time how well she looked.

Shortly after Bee's arrival, our friend Nancy Ritter called her family cardiologist, Dr. Robert Silverberg, and explained our situation. We were on the cusp of a cancer death and had no medical doctor on our side. As soon as Robert learned of our situation, he set up an appointment to see Chex that same day.

Nancy sent a limo over and Bud, the Ritters' faithful driver, helped Chex out of the house. He literally carried her down the stairs because she was so weak. Bee accompanied Chex to Dr. Silverberg's office. Because I had a commercial audition that afternoon, I met them there. I still had to make a living.

I found Chex in an X-ray room where she had just finished having X rays taken. We waited upstairs in an examination room until Robert came in and introduced himself. He asked me to come with him for a minute. In the sanctum of his office he said, "I was really hoping that I would be able to uncover some error in the Mexican clinic's diagnosis; some misinterpretation of the X rays. But they were right. Her lungs are totally metastasized with cancer. There really is nothing that can be done."

"How long?" I asked. He said that he didn't believe in giving time estimates because there was no way to know. But he guessed about six weeks.

We went in to talk to Francesca and Bee. Chex never asked for a prognosis and chose to address more practical concerns. She described her breathing problems and Robert immediately prescribed oxygen. He recommended that we talk to some home care specialists and hospice programs and gave us a few referrals. After he wished us well and promised to drop by to check up on her, we went home and began the business of dying.

I called hospices the next day. Cedars was my first call, but the receptionist put me on hold so I hung up. I have a real aversion to being put on hold. It took a few more calls before I finally came upon Home Healthcare. A lovely woman named Leslie Claire Fuller, who was full of life and compassion, answered the phone. I knew she would be the one. After Leslie agreed to come out and examine Chex, I told Chex that I had arranged for a hospice nurse. Chex's initial reaction was concern about some stranger taking over, but I reassured her that we would maintain control over the situation.

Bee remained with us for the duration and her arrival signaled the beginning of the Draper onslaught. This was the most challenging and rewarding phase of Chex's death. You see, the Drapers are a magnificent family, but they're very different from the Linkes. The Linke family operates independently. I always thought that we were like a four-car garage. The Drapers' lives are so intertwined, however, that they are much more like a plate of spaghetti. As soon as the word went out, they descended on Michael Avenue.

Bill, her dad, came out from New York; Willy, her brother, and his future wife, Terese, came from Colorado; and her sister, Maggi, came down from Mount Shasta. Bee stayed in the house with us while the rest of them moved into a nearby motel.

The Draper presence provided an environment for a rich experience. We loved and needed having her family there, but Chex and I vowed to have some private time for ourselves and our three children each day. It was important that the five of us maintain our own identity in the midst of all our visitors. It was like living in a Eugene O'Neill play.

There was one incident that I recall involving a yellow bell pepper imported from Holland at a cost of approximately $5.99 a pound. After I cut it up, Bee got on my case about being wasteful and leaving a little of the yellow meat on the stem. It was an acupressure point of anger for me.

"Look, Bee, this is a very difficult period and I think we have to be very honest with each other about our anxiety. This is not about how I cut my yellow bell pepper from Holland which I bought myself. This is about your daughter, my wife, who is dying. Let's be very clear about that. If we're going to make it

103

through this together, we need to give each other room to breathe without dumping on each other."

Chex and I decided to set up our home almost like a hospital with set visiting hours. We didn't want people to just come and hang out. I took on the main nurse's duty, which meant being on call from morning till late at night. Willy and Terese agreed to split the night shifts and came at 11:00 P.M. each night and were on call until the next morning. We created our own medication charts. We organized ourselves and worked together as a quasi-home medical team.

Each day was a marathon. In the midst of ongoing patient care and home death preparations, we still had to maintain a daily "normal" routine for the kids.

Chex was loved by many. As soon as people learned how sick she was, they started to arrive from all parts of the country. I am convinced that everybody who came to visit left with an individual life lesson forged by the alchemy of a final good-bye to someone they've loved. Everyone's private time with Chex was special to her, but was also taxing to her failing energy. There were even times when she was unable to cope with the effervescent level of energy from our children. I judiciously monitored her physical well-being and would clear the room when need be.

Everybody wanted to help. After a while, I started to take them up on their offers, and my standard request was for Thai food. I thought that the spicy quality of Thai cuisine would prevent me from coming down with a cold. You wouldn't believe how much horrible Thai food I wound up eating.

One woman persisted in her offer to help out. I finally asked her to find a Braun coffee glass decanter replacement. My original carafe had suffered a premature demise due to the overwhelming number of coffee-drinking visitors. It was truly the bottomless pot. I gave her twenty dollars and the name of an appliance store that carried them. That was the last I saw of her or my twenty dollars until the day of the memorial.

Lucinda, Chex's close friend from Sarah Lawrence College, arrived on crutches in a full leg cast. Torn ligaments from a skiing accident didn't stop her from maneuvering the thirteen steps upstairs to our bedroom. Lucinda bought Chex a portable stereo and music tapes after Chex mentioned that she missed hearing music.

Our Boulder, Colorado, friend and spiritual mentor, Myron, came three times. He and Chex prayed and talked and planned the memorial. He agreed to play the piano, and together they chose the music.

Nancy Ritter and Ry Hay took over some of the nursing shifts and stayed well into the night. My sister, Nanci, and her husband, Steve, shopped, helped with the kids, and provided an endless amount of support.

Glenda, Tara, Zena, cousins Will and Bobsey, and other devoted friends too numerous to mention here were all an integral part of the experience. They brought old pictures, crystals, and religious and spiritual artifacts, recounted past times, and laughed and cried together. It had all the earmarks of a reunion except that upstairs, above the din, was a dying Chex.

In an attempt to harness all this loving support and good intentions, we held a healing meditation for Francesca. Fifty people bursting with energy gathered in our living room one Sunday and prayed for a miracle. Gordon Spitzer, a hypnotherapist with whom Chex had been working, led the prayer session. I was astonished by the amount of love that rose up through the floor into the bedroom where I sat with a dozing Chex. Peace descended upon the house during those thirty minutes, and when it was over, everyone walked out in quiet reflection.

Our home had taken on a Jekyll/Hyde persona. Downstairs, it was Linke Hotel. Kids played, the TV blared, food was served, and life moved on. Upstairs, it was quiet, subdued, and shadowed in death. The stairs bridged the two worlds.

False Exit

"Paul, I think tonight's the night....I'm sorry, guys."

I don't know if it was due to the grains and greens diet, the colonics, the juices, or the vitamin supplements, but Francesca didn't have a lot of pain. She did struggle to breathe, however, which caused her great anxiety. As an asthmatic child, her worst fear was lung cancer and she now lived out that nightmare. Dr. Silverberg prescribed a very mild tranquilizer that really helped her to relax.

Francesca continued to take her Hoxsey tonic and male hormone injections. These shots of "bull balls" were one aspect of her treatment with which I couldn't deal. I'm not afraid of needles, but I was very uncomfortable with the idea of puncturing her skin. Our neighbor Mary Ann kindly gave her the injections. She had in the past given shots to her horses and was willing to do it.

The tranquilizers relaxed her, but the male hormones sexually aroused her. Ironic, isn't it? So much of my rage had centered around her not making love to me enough between babies and her illness. And now, just as I was coming to terms with her leaving, she was as horny as when we first met. Another one of God's karmic jokes, I guess.

The only pain medication we had on hand was Tylenol with codeine, which she only started to take toward the very end. Dr. Silverberg also prescribed oxygen. Every day I placed my order, and rather large men from a hospital supply company would arrive with enormous green canisters. I always feared that one of them would break or that the regulator wouldn't work, but they never failed us.

Once the home hospice routine was set up and running, most of the days blended together with a sameness in routine. There was, however, one particularly memorable night, a relatively quiet Saturday evening on Michael Avenue about four weeks before Francesca died. Her dear friend Myron was visiting from Colorado. He brought her small framed photographs of St. Francis of Assisi and Paramahansa Yogananda, which he placed around her. He sipped Scotch and constantly reassured her that these spiritual guides were in her presence.

I was downstairs chopping vegetables, a favorite "off duty" preoccupation, when Myron came into the kitchen to inform me that Francesca believed the end was near. I dropped my knife and abandoned my vegetables to rush upstairs to her side.

"Paul, I think tonight's the night," she said. I asked, "Are you sure?" She replied, "Yes. You'd better call everyone. I feel so tired."

I immediately put out the word via my prearranged "phone tree." Friends were assigned to call specific people who in turn had others to call. It was the only feasible way to reach the myriad of friends in a short period of time. "If you want to see her one last time, you'd better get here soon," I urged.

Myron and I quickly set up her "deathbed" scene. We placed her crystals around the room, lit candles, and played New Age composers on the stereo before settling in to wait for the "moment at hand."

By midnight our bedroom was filled to the rafters with family and friends. Bill Draper was the only one who hadn't arrived yet. I had telephoned him in New York and he promised to hop the first available flight. We all knelt, prayed, and listened to the tapes as Francesca prepared for her final journey. An hour passed and nothing happened. By 2:00 A.M., still nothing had happened, and there was a growing restlessness in the air. We watched intently and waited for her final moment to occur. Our candle-lit bedroom flickered with the images of her New Age funeral bier. Flowers, children's drawings, photos of everyone, healing stones, crystals, and tired bodies were crowded everywhere.

At 4:00 A.M., the vibes in the room were thick with death. Everyone moved closer to her as the moment seemed to have finally arrived. Bee held Chex's hand and stroked her forehead. Myron led everyone in prayer, Pachelbel's Canon played in the background, Maggi wept, and I marveled at the tableau. It was beautiful and artful. She was leaving us and we were all there. There was a distinct peacefulness in the room. Francesca came to consciousness and commented, "That was so close," then closed her eyes again.

At dawn Francesca's eyes popped open, as if from sleep, and gazed around the room at all the familiar faces. Chagrined, she sighed. "I'm sorry, guys. I guess I was wrong. It's not time yet. Thanks anyway." She looked remarkably refreshed while the rest of us looked like a group of "boat people" in need of rescuing. Actually, she was depressed about having to face another day of dying. Maggi brought a quote from Stephen Levine's *Who Dies?* to Francesca's attention that seemed to describe the moment: "Survival is highly overrated."

Later, Francesca recounted an out-of-body experience that was similar to the one discussed by Shirley MacLaine in *Out on a Limb.* Chex claimed she left her body and soared into the heavens above, but remained attached to her body by a silvery cord. When she bemoaned the fact that the cord hadn't snapped, I reminded her that we are not in control of such things.

I told her, "There will be a moment that will be your last and then there will be no more. Let's not rush it. It'll be soon enough." We laughed about the previous night's "false exit" and how hilarious it now appeared in the morning light. When her moment of death did arrive, I remember thinking back on this particular night and realized how premature we'd been and how different her final exit actually was.

Garden Story

"I'm so sick of this room...I want to see my garden again."

About three weeks before her death, Chex expressed a desire to spend some time in her garden. She had been bedridden for almost five weeks and felt claustrophobic. I initially resisted the idea. Her last attempt to get out of bed had been a failure. She had tried to join me for our Friday night TV ritual, "Miami Vice," but was too weak to make it downstairs and required the sustenance of her portable oxygen tank to get back to bed.

Getting her out into the garden was a major task. Chex was now hooked up to an oxygen tank twenty-four hours a day. The five-foot, septic green twin tanks and other medical equipment had turned our bedroom into a makeshift hospital suite. Not only was I concerned about how we would get both her and the oxygen outside, but I worried whether the effort would sap too much energy from her.

Her mom was very much in favor of the idea. "Some fresh air would really do her good," she persisted. Bee and I mildly debated over the proposed excursion until Chex's gentle voice stopped us.

"I'm so sick of this room. I'd really like to go outside. I want to see my garden again."

The family mobilized and got everything set up in the backyard while Willy and I carried her downstairs in a chair. She was attached to a portable tank to provide oxygen on the way to the

111

garden. As soon as we got her situated in a lounge chair under the peach tree, we switched over to the main tanks. I had discovered that the large tanks used in the bedroom had extremely long extension cords, and we were able to drop a mask out of the window and down into the backyard. With everything in place, we all pulled up chairs and gathered around her.

Chex cried at the sight of all the beautiful plants and flowers. Bee, an award-winning organic gardener, had been exercising her green thumb and the now-coming-into-bloom garden had never looked better. Francesca was surrounded by calla lilies, birds of paradise, roses, jasmine, orange and plum blossoms. We all took in the colors and fragrances of early spring, and she thanked her mom for doing such a great job. We had a garden party that was filled with lively conversations intermingled with moments of silence and herbal tea.

A soft breeze blew that afternoon, the same particular soft breeze that had always been present at significant times of our lives. It was at our wedding in Paradise Cove. It reappeared at Ryan's baptism on Venice Beach and at many times along our path. I even felt its gentle breath on my neck at Willy's wedding to Terese months after Chex was gone. It's a breeze that I still feel once in a while.

Jasper and Ryan arrived home from school and were surprised and delighted to find their mother outside. Little Rose crawled around on the grass and tried to climb up on Francesca. Bee served tea, Willy and Terese took pictures, and Bill sketched and told some of his delightful, witty stories. Maggi and Chex engaged in a sisterly talk while I sat quietly and kept watch over Rose.

We all had a wonderful time, and as it turned out, it was her last good day. When the afternoon sun faded, the breeze turned cool and Chex wanted to go back upstairs. We hoisted her up and carried everything back up to the bedroom.

Once settled in her bed, she thanked us all and mused on the afternoon. She had perceived a living message from Mother Nature in her garden. Winter was going out, spring was coming in, and life would go on.

Once again, Francesca had become our teacher. How does a terminal patient know when to stop the fight and surrender? Fighting, denial, and a will to live are all a part of overcoming a catastrophic illness and getting well. There is a point, however, when the struggle gets in the way and it's time to let go. Chex had fought hard and long for her life, but she had now crossed the threshold. She had found acceptance in her impending death and now tried to help the rest of us to do the same.

Letters to Chex

"Thank you for being my mom."
"Brava Francesca."

L eni Wildflower was by now a great ally. She came over every so often to answer our questions, and her arrival was always at the right time. Chex talked about what she was feeling and what her thoughts were, and Leni always had great advice and support to offer.

Leni's most valuable contribution to us was to get Jasper to sit down and express his feelings in a farewell letter to his mom. Because he couldn't yet write, Jasper dictated his thoughts, which Leni wrote out in longhand.

> *Dear Mom, I'll miss you when you go to heaven. But you'll be with me in my heart. I'm sorry you have to go. Thank you for being my mom. Love, Jasper.*

I watched from the bottom of the stairs as my little six-year-old boy took his expression of love up to his mom. I stood in the hallway and peeked in and watched him hand it to her. She read it and burst into tears. Chex grabbed for him and they held on to each other and cried. To Jasper, this letter is a tangible piece of his mom. It's something that they held on to together at the same time. It is now in his memory book, which he created with the help of his play therapist, Sally Reed, to serve as a place to put his love for his mom.

Jasper and Ryan covered the fireplace mantel in the bedroom with drawings for their mother. Jasper was in his "maximum butterfly period" at the time. In retrospect, isn't it interesting that that was the image which filled his head? The butterfly, transformed from a cocoon, is born out of death.

Inspired by Jasper's gesture, Bee also composed a note of thanks and love to her oldest daughter. It was very late one night when she came into the bedroom. After commenting on how Jasper shouldn't be the only one to write a letter, Bee sat on the floor and read hers to Chex.

> *March 22 '86—Dearest one, I love you with the greatest tenderness and humbleness through all your joys and sufferings. They have always given me comfort and courage. I am very proud of you. Even in your agonies, you have seldom complained and had the courage of your convictions making you a very total woman. Brava Francesca! From Mums.*

Francesca was very still. Her mom hugged her, grabbed both of Chex's hands and kissed them. Bee, whose face was etched in pain and acceptance, knelt and ministered to her. Across the dimly lit room, the image of Michelangelo's Pieta came to mind as I watched Bee lovingly hold her dying daughter and quietly pray.

The day after Francesca died, the Ritter family came over to the house. I walked out onto the front lawn to greet them. Carly, their four-year-old daughter, handed me a card that she had made. She had drawn a star in crayon and had Nancy write an inscription for her: "I want to say I love Chex and I want this star to make you happy."

116

A year after her death, Jasper wrote another letter to his mother in heaven as part of his ongoing play therapy.

Dear Mommy, I feel sad because you died. I look at your pictures on my dresser. I saw your picture and think "I miss you." I want you to know I am 7 now. And I learned how to cook eggs and sometimes I help my dad cook pancakes. I play the piano now. From, Jasper.

In retrospect, it is interesting to note the significance of these letters. At the time, they helped the authors cope with losing Francesca. With the passage of time, they help to keep her memory alive.

These written memories are even more poignant today and continue to be meaningful. To me, they are emotional photographs that captured an essential chord of the time.

Conversations She Was Dying to Have

"I love you, Chex..."
"I love you more."

I didn't know anything about dying. It had always been in the movies. It was *The Pride of the Yankees* or *Terms of Endearment* or Riff getting stabbed at the end of act i in *West Side Story.* Now it was a part of my life. I was shocked by the truth of it, amazed by the humor to be found in it, and shaken by the profound sadness of it all.

I had never thought that dying could mean my thirty-seven-year-old wife, tucked under the sheets and propped up on pillows, saying with a smile, "Paul, I just want to thank you for all those great orgasms you gave me. I wish I'd been a little wilder for you, Paul."

"Hey, Chex, you were the best."

Five weeks before she died, I found her in the bathroom leaning up against the doorjamb. I rushed to her aid because she was trembling, in obvious distress.

"What is it, Chex? What's the matter?"

"What will I tell Jasper?" she cried. "Tell me. What will I tell him?"

At that precise moment, our six-year-old boy ran in and looked up at his mom and dad in that horrible moment of their

119

lives. We three rushed together into an awkward triangular embrace, tripping and falling over one another onto the shag rug mat next to the tub. I listened as she explained, "Jasper, honey, you know how I've always told you that I was going to get well? And how after I got well we'd all go to Hawaii to celebrate?"

There was excitement in his face as he nodded in whole-hearted agreement.

"Honey, I may not get well. I'm trying, I'm really trying. I'm fighting every day. You and Ryan are such good boys, staying quiet to help Mama get her rest, but sweetheart, I may not get well."

An hour later I found an angry and exasperated Francesca in our bedroom. "Goddamnit," she said, weeping. "I am such a fool. Who did I think I was, anyway? Why didn't I listen to them?"

"Stop it, don't do this to yourself, Francesca. Honey, you have shown more courage than I could ever hope to display. You made the choices that you had to make at the time you needed to make them. Don't beat yourself up now."

One of my more powerful, emotional memories is that of my mother's last visit with Francesca. My mom had a very difficult time accepting Chex's illness. She had survived a benign brain tumor herself and couldn't reconcile the fact that it was Francesca who was dying and not her. She was so upset that she would hang up the phone whenever I called. Close to the end, she decided to come up for a visit. This was no mean feat considering her wheelchair-bound state and the thirteen steep, steps up to the bedroom.

Somehow we managed to get her up to Francesca's bedside, where I watched the two most important women in my life say their good-byes. After expressing thanks for her grandchildren, my mom leaned forward and said, "I want to thank you for helping my son to become a man."

Another particularly poignant good-bye occurred when our midwife, Vi, came to pay her respects. They wept as Vi thanked Francesca for all she had learned about birthing from her. Coming from a woman who had facilitated over four hundred births, it was the ultimate acknowledgment from one woman to another.

One afternoon I walked into our bedroom, looked at her lying there, and said, "Goddamnit, Francesca, this is so unfair. You're going to get to die and go off to be at peace. I'll be stuck here alone with three kids to raise all by myself. I can't do it, Francesca. I can't handle it. I just can't do it."

She looked up at me, smiled, and with absolute succinctness said, "But Paul, you're already doing it."

I broke down and cried. This was the first time that I'd really let my emotions out. She held me and started to cry herself. Together we sobbed inconsolably. Suddenly, struck by the high drama in our lives, we burst out laughing. We were literally laughing and crying at once. The mood in the room lightened. I never before understood how fine a line stood between tears and laughter. It was yet another unexpected episode in the irony of life.

One evening, we were sitting together when she asked, "Paul, tell me, have you thought about who you're going to go out with after I'm gone?"

Shocked, I quickly replied, "No! I can't say that I have."

Determined to pursue this line of conversation, Chex continued. "Well, I expect you to wait at least three months out of respect. But you're a young man with children. You need a woman around here. I wondered if maybe you had considered any candidates?"

"What is this, Chex, an election year?" I laughed. "I've been kind of busy nursing you, honey."

"Have you thought about going out with Nora?"

"Nora?" I shrieked. "Why are you trying to set me up with Nora?"

"Well," Chex counseled. "Nora is Ryan's nursery school teacher. She's very good with kids, and do you want to know something, Paul? I have always thought that Nora had a sneaker for you."

I thought about all the women whom I had mentally lusted after during my marriage. One woman came to mind. "Well," I slowly offered, "what about Beth?" You see, I always had a major sneaker for Beth.

She thought for a moment. Her expression narrowed. "Well, you know, Beth is pretty heavy, Paul. Why not Lucinda? She'd love to have some kids."

Suddenly, I looked at Francesca, "Wait a minute, honey, stop. I'm sorry. There's no way I can discuss my next relationship while you're still here with me."

She looked at me and very seriously said, "You're right. In fact, on second thought, you'd better wait six months."

We hugged and within a few minutes she dozed off. As I watched her sleep, I was touched by how remarkable my wife truly was. Even though she was dying, she was still concerned about my future well-being.

I came home early one morning after dropping the kids off at their respective schools to prepare for another day of nursing: there was oxygen to be ordered, hospice paperwork to be filled out, a grocery run to be completed, phone calls to be returned, and feet to be massaged. In a household with three children, life still had to go on. I took a break and went up to sit with Francesca as she sipped her Hoxsey tonic.

"You know what I realize, Chex?" I said. "We're working day after day toward your home death. All the preparations...it's just like the times we got ready for a home birth. Except this time, we're going to lose one in the process."

She smiled sadly. "I just wish it would happen. Why is it taking so long?"

"Believe me, it'll happen soon enough. Think of time as thread passing through the eye of a needle. There will be a point when you'll cross through it and be gone forever. Don't rush it."

Her waning days were a palette of emotions. Some laughter. Some tears. Some silence. I felt extremely close to her in those rich, quiet moments. In this serenity, everything seemed okay.

Late one afternoon Francesca suddenly looked at me. "Paul, there's something I have to know. Did you ever cheat on me?"

Now, talk about being put on the spot! In the moment of her question, my mind drifted back to the first time that she and I had ever made love. Afterward, she said, "Paul, do you realize what we just did? When we made love like that, do you realize that we created a bubble of light that surrounds us and binds us together. If we are faithful and only make love to each other, the more energy we'll create, the more light we'll fuse into our bubble, the more luminescence we give off, and the more we'll be bound together."

For ten years I had walked around this planet surrounded in all this light, convinced that if I strayed even *one* time it would be like taking a pin and pricking a hole in the bubble of light, allowing all the light to leak out onto the ground. I looked into those beautiful blue eyes and said, "No, Chex, I never cheated on you."

She smiled and nodded off. In that late afternoon light, in the silence as she began to sleep so peacefully, I finally understood the payoff for my fidelity.

On Rosie's first birthday, March 24, 1986, Francesca was very ill, and I was convinced that the only reason she was still with us was to defy Dr. Karlin and his words about making it to that one-year point. At 8:00 A.M. I brought Rosie into the bedroom and said, "Chex, honey, you know what day this is? It's Monday. It's the twenty-fourth. It's Rosie's birthday. You made it."

She looked up at me and smiled. "I can't believe it. I can't believe it." She said it with slow, slurred speech.

Later that afternoon as I walked out of the bedroom, I suddenly looked at her. "I love you, Chex."

Every time I left our bedroom in that final ten weeks of our life together, I always left her with the words "I love you, Chex."

I feared she might slip away while I was gone and wanted to leave her with that thought. Even if I went to the bathroom or changed Rosie's diaper or went downstairs for a cup of coffee, I never left her without saying, "I love you, Chex."

Frankly, I think Francesca had had it with all those announcements of affection because one morning, on my way to get the sports page, I turned and said, "I love you, Chex." She half smiled. "I...love...you...more," she gasped.

That was our final conversation.

Home Death

"It's time, Francesca...It's time to let go."

O n the night before Francesca died, Dr. Silverberg made a house call. He came to see Chex and, most important, to keep us legal. In the state of California, if you haven't been seen by a medical doctor within thirty days of your demise, an autopsy is mandatory by law. This kind doctor came to our home on his night off and brought his two sons, who waited in the car for him.

After Robert peeked in on Chex, he came down the stairs to where the family had gathered and simply said, "The breathing pattern that she's exhibiting is called stove-type breathing. This means she has thirty-six to forty-eight hours left. Right now, my main concern is that she's suffering from dehydration. She can't swallow, and I'm afraid that dehydration will take her before the cancer does. It's extremely painful and very unnecessary. Here's what I suggest: I want to get an IV unit to hydrate her and make her more comfortable. I'm not trying to prolong her life, I'm just trying to improve the quality of her final hours. A registered nurse is needed to run this equipment. I know that you've wanted to nurse her on your own, and you've done a great job, but I'm asking you to please untie my hands now. Let the professionals take over."

There was a palpable tension at the bottom of the stairs where everyone had alighted. It's funny. I don't remember the specifics of what anyone said, but I do remember that everyone's fears emerged from the shadows. A debate about nothing ensued. Perhaps because we had come so far together, we were able to express our fears and recognize our anxiety. We realized that we couldn't change the outcome and were experiencing the inevitability of the process. We all finally agreed that he was right. It was time for a nurse to come in and help us.

"Look, I'll order a nurse to start tonight. Give yourselves a break. Go out to dinner or go to a movie. I'll have an IV delivered in the morning. Also, there's one thing you should understand. When you're in the room with Francesca, I want you to keep talking to her, okay? The last sense to go is hearing, so it's very important that you all keep talking to her right through the end."

He ordered a nurse and the Drapers dispersed while I went upstairs to be with Francesca.

I sat in the dimly lit bedroom with her and thought how hard we had tried to guard our private time. And yet our home had become Grand Central Station. There in the darkness, I spent my final quality moments with her. The whirlwind of the last ten weeks was over. All that remained was a peaceful quiet in our home and serenity in our hearts. We had, after all, come to a place of love and healing.

Chex laid in a semicomatose state with her eyes not quite open, but not quite closed. In the final seventy-two hours of her life, there had been a rapid transition in her physical condition. It seemed as if she had wasted away overnight. Her eyes had filmed over, which dimmed their blueness. Her teeth were coated. Her skin was ashen. It was hard to tell if she knew what was going on or not.

The peace was shattered by the phone ringing. It was the registered nurse who was scheduled to work that night. She told me that her sixteen-year-old daughter had failed to return home from a date and she wouldn't be able to come because she was worried about her. She said she was sorry, but there was nothing that she could do. I hung up the phone and looked over at the TV clock radio that "CHiPs" had given me so many Christmases before. It was 10:45 P.M. I was angry that she had left me in the lurch. Chex couldn't be alone and everyone had gone off assuming that the nurse would be there. Exhausted, I knew I couldn't stay up all night with her. Fifteen hours a day for nearly ten weeks had taken its toll on me and I desperately needed my rest. I was in a panic until I suddenly remembered an offer of help from my neighbors, the O'Briens. They had said that if I ever got stuck, they would gladly sit with her. I called and Mary Ann agreed to come over and sit with her from 11:00 P.M. until 2:30 A.M. Her husband, Mike, would relieve her then and stay until dawn.

Once Mary Ann settled down with Chex, I was able to get my wearied body between the sheets. I looked over across the room and fell into a sort of dreamlike semisleep that was filled with a vision. It was a 360-degree panorama of clouds, just like the Sensurround film exhibit at Disneyland. Everywhere I looked, there were clouds. At the center of these clouds was a peaceful spot. It reminded me of a time when I had driven across Arizona at midnight under a full moon. It was the same sense of peace that lingered in the air that night. I was aware of a golden light that emerged from behind the clouds. It was everywhere. Much more immense and infinite than anything I had ever imagined. It shot out rays of golden light that pierced the clouds. It all came together and interconnected in the center of this peace.

I was stunned. This was *our source* and I believed that it was Francesca's way of telling me that it was okay to let her go because she was going to a far, far better place.

I awoke with a start to find Michael O'Brien, FBI agent, sitting by Chex's side. With a coffee mug in one hand, he was reading a book by flashlight while listening to all-night talk radio on a headset. It was a bizarre image to behold. The juxtaposition of God and Larry King boggled my mind. I knew I wouldn't go back to sleep. I asked, "Mike, do you want some more coffee?"

Downstairs, I fired up the Braun Aromaster and made twelve cups of the Rose blend, half-French, half-Colombian dark roast. Bleary-eyed, I watched the dark liquid drip into the clear glass carafe until I heard Francesca moan and cry. I bolted upstairs. At the top of the stairs stood a pajama-clad Jasper. He was frozen in place with his eyes transfixed on the half-open door to our bedroom while he listened to his mother groan and murmur, "Mama, mama."

Home death means not hiding from anything. Home death is grief before breakfast. Home death is breaking down and crying on your way to pee in the morning because you pass by your dying wife to get to the bathroom. Home death is having your children, the whole human beings that they truly are, fully participate in the experience. I grabbed my little boy and hugged him as tightly as I could. We went into the bathroom, where I gave him a drink of water and then tucked him back into his bunk bed. I returned to the bathroom and opened the mirrored medicine cabinet to find Tylenol with codeine, the only pain medication she was on. Overwhelmed with frustration and fatigue, I stood there and furiously ground it up. She couldn't swallow anymore so I had to mix it with a dime-sized pool of water, the least amount of liquid possible. I injected the mixture into the back of her throat with a syringe and prayed that her throat lining would absorb the medication. I cursed at how barbaric it was.

I sipped coffee with Mike O'Brien throughout the rest of the night. Around 6:00 A.M., Mike stood up, gathered his belongings, strapped on his gun, and went off to chase bank robbers for the day.

At 6:20 A.M. the full light of day had filtered into the room. I looked at Francesca and knew she was going to die that day. Every moment got so *big*. I looked out a window into the backyard and gazed down on the apple tree. Francesca's spirit appeared in the branches of the tree. It looked like a cameo portrait. She wore her favorite serape and her blondish-brown hair flowed in the gentle breeze. Her eyes sparkled blue and alive. I thought I was seeing her spirit leave her body and couldn't believe it. I looked back at her, but her face bore no witness to what I thought had just occurred.

I got on the phone at 8:00 A.M. to beg the hospice nurse for morphine. At nine, an RN finally appeared with an IV unit. She hooked it up and Francesca seemed to be much more comfortable. Our friend Steven Keats arrived around ten with a pain injection that he had picked up from Beverly Hills Medical Center at the doctor's request. The nurse administered it, and this brought Francesca some more relief.

The morphine didn't arrive until 11:00 A.M. and the paperwork took thirty minutes to complete. Finally, Francesca received her first injection of morphine, half of what the doctor had prescribed.

Five minutes later, as I stood by the water bed and talked to the RN and the Hospice nurse about what I should expect, I turned around and looked at Francesca. Her face had rapidly lost all color. I didn't know people could lose color that quickly. It was as if her face was a clear blue cloudless sky with a quickly encroaching, horrible black storm suddenly moving across. Her life plug had been pulled out and she was draining away. I anxiously brought it to the nurses' attention. "What's going on? What's happening with her?"

The older nurse said, "She's going."

I snapped at her, "Go get her family. Please just go downstairs and get the family for me."

I turned again and found that Francesca's face had taken on an unearthly glow. I rushed to her side, pulling up a chair to sit. I had promised to be there at the instant of death to help her make the final crossing. I hadn't left my house in ten days, the moment was at hand, and I was ready to fulfill my promise. In an attempt to do my Stephen Levine conscious-dying best, I leaned in and whispered some final words of encouragement in her ear.

"I'm right here, Chex. I know you can hear me. I want you to know that you are doing a great job. You are doing such good work. I'm so proud of you. Easy, honey. Soft Belly, Chex. It's time, Francesca. It's time to let go and let God...Your body doesn't work for you anymore. So cast it aside, fly up to the sky, easy, honey. Don't resist it. Let go. Let God open your heart, honey. Let it wash over you like a gentle summer rain. Go to the light. Seek the light. Easy. You're doing good, you are doing such great work. I am so proud of you. You are so fantastic. Good girl. Soft Belly, Chex. Here comes your mom now and your dad's right with her. And here comes Terese too. See, we're all right here with you, honey. You're not alone. You've got us all here. You've given us all so much in your lifetime. Even now. In the moment of your death, you're giving each of us the gift of life. Easy, honey. We all talked last night like you asked, and I want you to know that we all release you. You have our permission. It's okay. You're so beautiful, Francesca. Honey, I want you to know that I'm ready. I really am. I swear to you that I am going to be the greatest dad for those kids. You don't have to stick around anymore for me. I can handle it. Easy, honey. I love you, Chex. I'll love you forever. Go to God, honey... Go to God... Just let... go."

I was totally aware and completely focused on each and every moment. I secretly hoped that at the critical moment, if I looked deep enough into those beautiful blue eyes, I'd perhaps grasp a glimpse of the beyond. But all I saw was her breathing become increasingly labored and irregular while her body fought for life. Finally, Francesca took what turned out to be her last breath and was gone.

Chex's mouth opened, her jaw went slack, there were no more breaths. She was gone. After a moment or so, a single tear formed in her left eye. As the drop rolled down her cheek on its solitary journey, I wiped it away with my right forefinger and placed it in my mouth to savor her final gift to me.

We all sat quietly. We had reached the end of the journey. There was a very surreal quality to the noontime light that washed across the room in pale golden hues. Chex's garden was in full bloom and its rich fragrance wafted through the bedroom window. For a few minutes, no one uttered a sound. We were all deep in reflection about this profound experience. She was gone and we had all somehow been changed. I suddenly craved my children.

"Somebody get the kids please. Will somebody please get my children."

Just before she passed, my friend Steven had popped his head in the door to ask if I wanted the children brought up. I was so immersed in my coaching that I did not want to stop to respond. A few minutes after her death, three-year-old Ryan appeared. He looked at the scene, quickly made a beeline over to his Grandpa Bill, and climbed up onto his lap.

As soon as Jasper appeared, I grabbed him tightly and said, "Your mom's gone, honey. You see. She's with God now. It's okay, honey. I'll be there for you. I'll take good care of you. I'm not going anywhere, you hear me. I love you, my big boy."

I called the mortuary, as I'd been instructed to do, to inform them that she was gone. The woman on the phone told me how sorry she was to hear the news and then said, "Mr. Linke, when would you like us to come get her?"

"I don't know," I said. This was one aspect that I hadn't thought out. It was just like being pregnant, going to childbirth classes, and making preparations for the new arrival. No one ever tells you what to do with the baby *after* its birth. Francesca and I had worked toward the moment of her death, but now that it had occurred, I was left to deal with the result. I searched for an answer until I finally cleared my throat and said, "Well, tell me, how long do people usually take?"

"Well, Mr. Linke," she said. "Some people have us come right away and some people wait a day or two."

I hesitated. "I don't think I want to wait a day or two. How about three o'clock?" It sounded like a good time. I went out to the backyard to commune with Francesca's flowers.

Bee, Maggi, and all the rest of the women in the household took charge of moving Chex from the temporary hospital bed that we had fashioned by strapping a chair and ottoman together back onto the water bed. They dressed Chex in the gown she had chosen to be cremated in and collected all the crystals in the house.

As I stood in the backyard, Bee appeared with some scissors and began cutting some of Chex's daisies. I followed her inside and back upstairs. Francesca was laid out on the water bed atop our wedding quilt in her favorite gown, totally surrounded by crystals while her mother was busy placing the freshly cut flowers between her toes. I smiled to myself. Francesca would have loved this picture.

About twenty minutes later, her brother Willy arrived with a camera and took pictures of everything. I thought it was a trifle bizarre at the time, and today all those photos show is an ugly picture of a cadaver, a woman ravaged by cancer. However, if you had been in the room with us that afternoon, you would have experienced an energy that was present. There was a very special light in the room. It was something that no camera could capture, but it was real and it felt good to be with her.

I remember my dear father showed up in an hour with his two daughters from his second marriage. Neither girl would come into the room; they were too spooked out about a dead body. It meant a lot to me that my dad got there.

Friends and family gathered rapidly as the word went out. We all visited and enjoyed the time. At one point, everyone left me alone with Chex and I lay next to her on the water bed. I think everyone felt that I needed to have a private moment with her. I half expected a profound emotional experience as I lay there. But nothing happened—except that the phone rang. After what seemed to be an appropriate length of time, I called everyone back into the room.

Rosie climbed up on the bed, and everyone watched as she explored her mother's body. It appeared that she was trying to get a reaction from her. I thought that if other people ever knew about this, they'd find it a little macabre, but this tactile approach was probably Rose's way of coming to terms with her mom's death.

By three o'clock nearly everyone, except her best friend, Nancy, had arrived. I heard footsteps on the stairs and realized that the morticians had come to take her. But it was too soon and I realized that Nancy wouldn't get to see her unless I stalled for more time. I rushed out the bedroom door just in time to greet two brown-suited, brown-tied gentlemen at the top of the stairs who were peering into the bedroom. I said, "Look, can we go out into the backyard and talk?"

We went into the backyard and sat by my bonsai trees. Like bookends, the morticians sat there, cross-legged in stereo. My dear friend John Ritter was with us. John, who is a loving man, has a desire to always take care of things for his friends. He was there to help me. The morticians were instantly aware of the fact that a celebrity was with us. One of them turned and said, "Aren't you John Ritter?"

I thought, "God, isn't this amazing. My wife has just died and these guys are going to ask John for his autograph. This is totally inappropriate."

And I said, "Look guys, it's John Ritter. He's a very famous actor but right now he's here as my best friend. Could we not get into this, okay?"

The young mortician looked at me and said, "Mr. Linke, I hope you don't mind my asking but she looked so young, may I ask how she died?"

"She had cancer," I said.

"Cancer?" he said. "That's so sad."

"No," I said, "You don't understand what went on in our home. You see we had a conscious death experience. We had the opportunity, no, I should say we had the *privilege* to know that she was going to die, which allowed us to take advantage of the time that was left. You see, we took care of all of our business together. We cleaned it all up. We went into our psychological closets together. You want to know something, if you went into that closet right now and ran a white glove across its top shelf there would be no dust. We were immaculate in our closure. You want to know something, in this whole process, all Francesca and I could find was our love. No, this was the most beautiful thing, the most unbelievable experience I have ever been through."

The young mortician looked at me very askance and said, "You know something, Mr. Linke? You would do very well in our business."

"Now, this is totally bizarre," I thought. "My wife just died, she's laid out upstairs, and this guy is job-recruiting me! And what's worse is I'm an unemployed actor and I'm considering it!"

"Look," I said. "I know I told you 3:00 P.M., but her best friend, Nancy, hasn't made it yet. I wonder if you could go away and give me another hour?"

"Oh, I'm sorry, Mr. Linke. We'd love to help you, but we can't. We're very busy. It is a holiday weekend, you know."

"Yeah, I know, it's Easter weekend." The thought suddenly struck me that Francesca was born on Christmas Eve and died on Holy Thursday.

"I bet if you really put your minds to it, there is some solution you could come up with for me," I said, suppressing my irritation.

"Well, you see, the thing is, there's another van in the field, but he's picking someone else up, and I've got to go back with Bob here, and he's got to go home. I've got to mind the store, and well, there is one thing we could. But it would mean that she'd have to ride back with another."

"You mean there would be another body in the van with her?" I asked.

"That's right," he said quite delicately.

"Oh, that's great. Francesca would love company."

So I got my extra hour and Nancy made it over to the house to say her good-byes. At 4:00 P.M. on the dot, the second van pulled into the driveway and parked. Chex's new friend was inside. We were wheeling Chex out of the house when a big brouhaha ensued. Our housekeeper spoke in furious Spanish and made wild hand gestures. Someone finally understood that she was warning us that the body was leaving the house headfirst, which to her meant bad luck. She forced the poor mortician to back the gurney up the stairs and turn Francesca around so that she could leave feet first. We finally got her into the back of the van, and the mortician shut the gate. The van slowly backed out of the driveway and headed out of our lives forever. There were about forty of us on the front lawn that afternoon. We hugged each other, some waved good-byes, some cried, some laughed. "Good-bye, Chex."

Right then I learned that things are as true in death as they are in life. You see, when Francesca was alive, whenever we'd go anywhere, we would always get about a block away from the house and she'd always say, "Oh, Paul, honey, I'm sorry. Can we go back? I left my purse at home." "Oh, Paul, honey, I'm sorry, can we go back? I left the coffee maker on." "Oh, Paul, I'm sorry, honey. Can we go back? I left two of the kids at home."

The brown van was halfway down the street when someone hollered, "See you in the afterlife, Chex." At that instant, the van's taillights flashed red. It stopped, made a U-turn, came back up Michael Avenue, and pulled into the driveway and parked. I turned to everyone, "Geez, I wonder what she forgot *this* time?"

I had carefully arranged for the kids to be out of the house during all of this. As much a part of her illness and death as they were, I really did not want them to see their mother's body being taken from the house. I felt it was an unnecessary image for them to hold in their young minds. Some friends had taken them to a double feature. I was so nervous that they might show up in the midst of it all that I literally had sentries posted at both ends of Michael Avenue.

Once the van was finally on its way, we all went about the business of creating a home wake. I needed everyone around me and they all needed to be there. John and cousin Alla went out and brought back an incredible amount of Thai food, which we spread out on the table. Finally, good Thai food. We all ate, drank, and basically had an outrageous party together. The video of Francesca's last concert performance at the Powerhouse played in the living room. People walked around the house in search of memories. I held court in the bedroom, where the sweet smell of oxygen lingered in the air.

Later that night, my friends Dennis, Steven, and Andy took me to a Russian bathhouse for a svitz. It felt very ritualistic to sweat in a hot steamy room while old Russian Jews beat each other with eucalyptus leaves.

Steven stayed over in case I became upset in the middle of the night and needed someone to talk to. I appreciated it, even though I felt okay. I looked in on my sleeping children before climbing into my king-sized water bed. I stretched my legs out really wide and sensed the emptiness of the space all around me. I had begun the next phase of my life as a widower.

136

Jasper Canal Story

"Jasper, don't get wet."
"I won't, Paul. I promise."

When someone dies you're surrounded by love and attention. People call, write, send flowers, and make lasagna that you hate. Who makes lasagna with zucchini pieces in it? I wasn't exactly Nathan Pritikin, after all, so I froze the lasagna. It ended up going bad due to a power failure, but I was left with a nice new Pyrex dish in the transaction.

The point is that soon everyone's attention revolves back to his or her own life. Five days after Francesca died, I decided to explore my single-dad-ness and take my kids to the beach. Of course, as soon as we arrived, they started to complain about why we hadn't gone to the Venice canals, which we had passed on the way, instead. I was in an inflexible mood, but they promoted, lobbied, and bitched until I finally caved in even though it was cold and getting late and I still had to shop for a "healthy" dinner.

Jasper and Ryan tore out of the car and were off like a shot before I had even had the chance to extract Rosie from her car seat. I looked over the top of the Peugeot and yelled for them to come back. They rushed back like two obedient little puppies with their tongues dangling out of the corners of their mouths. I issued the directive, "Jasper, stay away from the water." Jasper is an Aquarius with a remarkable ability to find any body of water within a two-mile radius and fall into it. "Jasper, *don't get wet.* Do you hear me?"

"I won't, Paul." My kids call me Paul once in a while. "I promise."

They were off like a shot again while I got Rosie out of the car. I carried her and walked along. I stopped when I saw a Thai restaurant and thought back on Francesca's final weeks when I was obsessed with Thai food. I wondered if this restaurant served good Thai food and started to go inside to get a menu.

Something stopped me and I turned to check on the boys. A nice couple blocked my view while they oohed and ahhed over Rosie. I thanked them and looked over to Jasper in the distance. He was at the edge of the canal doing what could best be described as a kind of whirly-birdie right at the edge of the waterline. He was throwing his hands up and down, jumping around. I was seized with fear and about to call out to him when he tripped. For once in his life, he didn't fall in. This time he tumbled into Ryan and knocked *him* into the canal instead. My three-and-a-half-year-old fell facedown into the murky, brackish canal water.

I could see from ninety feet away that he was in trouble. His feet remained on the sidewalk where he had just stood, but his body was submerged underwater. His down vest had slipped over his shoulders and had turned into a restraint of sorts that prevented him from being able to pull himself up. He was drowning.

I rushed over to rescue him. I plunked Rosie down hard on her butt. A stranger came over to help me, and together we extricated Ryan from the canal. He was covered with muck, which he spat out of his mouth. Ryan started to cry from shock and the cold. All warmth had left the wintery day. I gathered up Rosie and herded the flock back to the car. As we walked, I grabbed Jasper at the base of his neck in a Vulcan grip.

"Goddamn it, Jasper. I told you to stay away from the water, didn't I? You didn't listen to me, did you? Your brother could be dead because of you. I am your father, Goddamnit. And when I tell you to do something, you're going to do it, you understand me? Now go to the car. I don't want to look at your face right now. When we get home I want you to go to your room. I don't want to look at your face until tomorrow, do you hear me. Fuck you, Jasper."

Hours later, back in our two-story Cape Cod house, Ryan was fully recovered. Squeaky clean from a bubble bath and wearing his favorite pajamas, he sat at the dining-room table and sipped hot chocolate. Ryan cast out pearls of wisdom to the room. "I could have drowned," he said innocently.

I went upstairs to talk to Jasper. I knocked on his door. "Jasper? Hey, Jasp. I'm sorry, honey. I'm sorry that I yelled at you and said those things to you. When I saw your brother in the water I was afraid he was going to die....If anything happened to any of you kids right now, I don't think I could live through that. My plate is full right now. Can you understand that? Jasper, I've been thinking. I don't think I yelled at you because you knocked Ryan into the canal and I don't think you're crying because I yelled at you. I think you're crying because your mom is gone and I yelled because I'm really angry about it. For some weird reason this was a way for you and I to help each other to get in touch with these feelings."

Ashes to Ashes

"Oh, my God, Ryan, look! You've got your mother all over your shoes!"

One of our many deathbed conversations concerned the final disposition of her body. "Paul, do you know what I'd really like? I'd like to be taken somewhere and simply have my body put in the dirt and covered up so I can return to Mother Earth and become one with her again."

"No coffin?" I asked. She shook her head no. "Wait a minute," I quickly interjected. "Don't you dare die before we talk about this, do you hear me? You cannot leave me with this request," I insisted. Everyone knows how sacred deathbed requests are.

I sat there and imagined myself looking for a county that would allow me to honor her wishes, to just dig a hole and stick her in the ground. "Chex, can't you just see me dragging you all over on various trains...you sitting there next to me and all the other passengers looking at us in horror? 'No, she's not sick, she's just dead. I'm trying to find a place to bury her.'"

She finally decided on cremation and asked if I would take her ashes to northern California and scatter them on Mount Shasta, an area considered by many to be a holy place. I promised I would.

To arrange for her cremation, I called several different funeral homes and entered into a whole new realm. I phoned the Neptune Society and got an answering service. I then called another company and got an answering machine. I finally connected with the Armstrong ("It's nice to be a member of the") Family and made all the arrangements. The staff instructed me to call after she died and they'd come and take her.

The Armstrong Family informed me that for an additional forty dollars, I could have my dearly departed's ashes delivered to my home. I figured the expense was well worth not having to make the trip. About ten days after she died, I got a phone call saying the ashes were ready and would be delivered that afternoon. I was told that Mr. Armstrong himself would be stopping by on his way home.

I looked out the window just as his white Plymouth pulled up. I opened the door before he could ring the bell. The kids were playing in the living room.

"Hi, I'm Bob Armstrong. I'm looking for Paul Linke."

"I'm Paul Linke," I said. His expression changed radically as his eyes shifted to the children playing in the background. He had assumed that he was delivering the ashes of an older person, someone who had lived a full life and passed on. It only took a moment before he realized that he was delivering a young woman's ashes. Tears welled up in his eyes as it registered that the box contained the cremains of my wife and that the children who were playing on the floor were motherless.

Before he brought the ashes inside, I directed my housekeeper to take the kids for a walk. As soon as they left, Bob Armstrong went to his car and retrieved a shoe box—sized, whitish cardboard box from out of his trunk. He walked back into the house, handed it to me, and proceeded to tell me how upset he felt. He explained that the situation had jolted his standard professional demeanor because he so strongly identified with me. We were about the same age and his wife was Francesca's age and they too had three children. He candidly admitted that if anything happened to them, he wouldn't be able to go on.

Often during the course of Francesca's illness and death, I had assumed the role of comforter. Many times, friends and visitors would come under the pretext of offering solace, only to wind up in need of comforting themselves. This time, I was offering solace to the mortician, a professional in death. I hugged him and he told me that he was anxious to get home to hug his wife and kids.

While waiting for the trip north, the ashes "lived" in various places around the house, including several closets and the garage. I diligently kept them out of the children's sight until the children's play therapist, Sally Reed, broached the subject.

Sally explained, "There is something the kids need to know, Paul. They don't understand what happened to their mother's body."

I was floored. They had come into the room after she died and saw her body. But when they returned from the movie, she wasn't there. They didn't get it. They knew she was dead but they didn't understand where the body was. Even though death had been explained to them, they weren't prepared for its practical aspects. As time passed, they grew more reluctant to bring it up. With Sally's help, we opened up a dialogue. I used the image of a big pizza oven to explain cremation. I reassured them that their mother's spirit was no longer in the body and that it didn't hurt her when it burned up. It was at this point that I brought up the ashes. When I asked if they wanted to see the box, they said yes. I brought it down and let the two boys hold it. Jasper commented on how heavy it was, and Ryan smiled as he hugged it. As soon as they had their moment with the box, they ran out to play. A great mystery had been so simply unraveled for them.

It's interesting to note that the one element in the whole home death experience that I tried to protect them from turned out to be the one great mystery they needed to solve. Perhaps our duty as parents isn't to "protect" children from instances like these, but to reassure them with the truth. It makes me wonder how many times we as parents think we are protecting our children when we are actually doing them a disservice. Kids know.

It wasn't until June of 1987 that I was able to fulfill my promise to Francesca. I drove a rental van up to Mount Shasta and parked the van where the road ended. Accompanied by Chex's sister, Maggi, Ryan and Jasper, we hiked up the mountain, carrying that funny white cardboard box. As we walked along, I realized it was time to confront the contents of the still-sealed container. Chex's good friend Myron had warned me at the memorial that there might be more than just ashes inside the box. He cautioned there might be bone fragments and "globules." Now, I didn't know what a globule was, but it sounded kind of gooey and clumpy and very intimidating.

After a short trek, I spied a beautiful little nestle of trees on the mountain slope and decided on it as the spot. We hiked over, and after spending a moment in quiet meditation, I dug a little hole. When I finished, I turned to my five-year-old Ryan, shook the ash-filled box, and asked, "Ryan, honey, what do you think is in this box?"

He thought for a long moment before offering his toothless grin and answer, "Eyeballs."

The tension thus being broken, I proceeded to open the box and pull out the clear plastic sack that held her remains. It wasn't weird, there weren't any eyeballs. It was just ashes and hard little bone fragments. I opened the sack and felt her. I took a little bit of the pumicelike remains and placed them into the hole. Jasper and Ryan both gingerly repeated the ritual.

I then grabbed a large handful and scattered them into the wind. The dust and ashes came to rest at the base of a tall redwood tree where a lot of tiny pink flowers were growing. The boys got caught up in the thrill of the moment. They were excited to scatter their dusty handfuls of her into the wind. They laughed as they threw handfuls to the left and the right. I stood back and watched.

After they were finished, I said, "Oh my God, Ryan, *look!* You've got your mother all over your shoes!"

I covered the hole and moved a big flat rock to demarcate the spot. Jasper and Ryan played on the mountainside while Maggi and I reminisced about Francesca. Her journey was finally complete and she was truly home at last.

Always in Our Hearts

"But if you die, Mom, how are you going to be there
for me, Mom?"

About three or four weeks before Francesca died, I walked into our bedroom one evening and found her with Jasper as they were finishing up a conversation. After she hugged and kissed him on the top of his little head, he jumped off the water bed and ran out of the room as if some great burden had been lifted off his shoulders. I asked what miracle she had just performed to raise his spirits so high.

"Well, Paul, I've been so worried about him ever since I told him that I might not get well, he has been so depressed. He was sitting on the floor, moping around when I said, 'Jasper, are you okay?'

"'No.'"

"'Want to talk about it?'"

"'No.'"

"'Is it because of me?'"

"'Uh-huh.'"

"'Jasper, I'll always be there for you.'"

"'But if you die, Mom, how are you going to be there for me, Mom?'"

"'Jasper, I will always be in your heart.'"

About two months after she died, I drove the boys to school early one morning. They had both opted to sit in the backseat, which qualified me as the chauffeur for the day. I watched their conversation in my rearview mirror. It was led by Jasper.

"Ryan, are you okay?"

"No."

"Want to talk about it?"

"No."

"Is it about our mom?"

"Yes."

"Ryan, don't you know...she's always in our hearts."

Thoughts on Grief

"So, Paul, what's new with you?"

G rief doesn't begin when someone dies. I had first learned this in the silence on the drive home from the Hoxsey Clinic on the day we learned Francesca's cancer had metastasized and she was terminal. I was reminded of this painful lesson on Jasper's sixth birthday, which was about six weeks before she died. Nancy Ritter and I had planned a joint birthday party at Disneyland for Jasper and her son Jason, whose birthday was one day earlier. Francesca was upset that we'd be gone all day and that she couldn't go.

On the way to Anaheim, I looked around in the van at my friends and all their children. Everyone was so upbeat, but I felt very alone. It suddenly dawned on me that this was a dress rehearsal for my future widowerhood. I felt an overwhelming sense of grief in the pit of my stomach and turned my head away as the tears flowed. I didn't want my friends to see how sad I was, and I certainly didn't want to spoil Jasper's day. Later when I looked at pictures taken of Jasper that day, I could see how sad he too had been. He didn't eat any birthday cake that day, nor for many years.

Another thought I have on grief is that it always comes up when you least expect it. In my case, it happened in the fall of 1986 on Jasper's first day at Crossroads Elementary School. Like many parents, I live vicariously through my children and the first day of school is a major event every year even for me. I still can't sleep the night before because my mind thinks back to all my first days of school and the nights before. My mother carefully shopped for my back-to-school clothes and meticulously laid them out at bedtime. As an overweight child, everything I wore was purchased in the "husky" section of a department store and only came in brown, charcoal gray, or blue. Every year, I was a dinner-sized fashion plate.

Fortunately, my kids are in good physical shape. I carefully laid out Jasper's outfit for his first day and was dead tired the next morning because I didn't sleep the whole night. At dawn I prepared his lunch and woke him at 6:20 A.M. for a power-packed high-carbohydrate breakfast. He was in a daze and didn't understand why he had to get ready for school so early. By eight o'clock, we were off to school. I parked and walked him across the street, proudly holding his little hand. As we entered the school grounds, I saw a group of mothers greeting one another. When I closed the gate, I saw more moms congregating in the courtyard. I looked around me and everywhere I looked, there were moms. And more moms. All moms...and me.

All of a sudden, I learned this lesson about grief. The truth is, you don't always see it coming. It's like a left hook that catches you by surprise, BOOM! Intense pain surged from my heart and I nearly broke down and cried right in front of my little boy. I stopped myself because I didn't want to taint his first day or ruin his experience. I rushed him into the classroom to divest myself of him so that I could go somewhere and weep. I literally pushed him through the door and fled to a dark place, where I cried nonstop for forty-five minutes over the fact that Jasper didn't have his mom there for him on his first day of school.

Part of this lesson in grief is that it dissipates as quickly as it arises. This was clear to me when I picked him up at 3:00 P.M. that day. I felt much better as I sat on the wall and waited for him to be dismissed. Thinking back over the morning, I decided that my grief had been like a tropical rainstorm that had rapidly appeared in a sudden cloudburst before moving on to its next destination. His classmates started to run by, but no Jasper. I finally asked his friend Jason where he was.

"Paul, hurry. Jasper fell down the stairs and hurt himself. He's at the bottom of the stairs. Hurry, Paul."

I ran over and found him at the bottom of thirteen concrete steps. He was in a heap crying convulsively.

I finished a cursory examination and determined that nothing was broken, all his limbs were intact, and there were no surface wounds. It then struck me what was going on. It was his first day of school without his mom, and he too was experiencing grief. As a six-year-old, he had no way to get in touch with these feelings and created a situation in order for them to come out. He needed to vent his tears.

Normally I always have something to say, but this was one time there was nothing I could say. All I could do was hold him closely and be there for him. After a while, I could feel his tiny fingers holding me back.

When someone dies, inevitably somebody will come up with the classic line, "Just make it through the first year and things will get better. All you've got to do is make it through the yearly milestones and the holidays."

This sympathetic offering of hope got its first serious challenge at Christmas. Francesca's birthday was December 24 and she would have been thirty-eight. It was a loaded day for me, but I decided not to run or hide from it. Instead, I held a Christmas Carols Open House for my family, my friends, and their children.

The exterior of our Cape Cod house was not decorated since I had decided that we needed the lights inside instead. I hired a pianist and had sheet music printed. When the day arrived, it was unusually hot, even for southern California. It was almost ninety degrees when we gathered in a circle around Francesca's piano drinking hot chocolate. We sweated bullets as we sang songs of the season in memory of Francesca. There was one thing that I did for myself in honor of her birthday. I ordered a dozen sterling roses that were delivered to the house and I placed them atop the piano. The beautiful flowers took center stage as all those loving voices filled the room. It's become a tradition that we still do every Christmas Eve.

Later, after everyone went home to be with their families and their trees, and my kids were tucked in dreaming of Santa, I went upstairs to sleep. As I got halfway up the stairs, I suddenly remembered the sterling roses. I went back down, picked up the vase, carried it up the stairs, and placed it on the nightstand next to the bed. I stretched out on our king-sized water bed and tried to sleep. It was at the stroke of midnight, when Christmas Eve turned into Christmas Day, that I reached the lowest emotional point of the first year. I felt so alone. I had lost the flower in the garden of my life and wondered if love would ever bloom for me again.

The first anniversary of Francesca's death coincided with the opening of a play that I was starring in. My role was that of a sociopathic serial killer. The important aspect of the play was that it allowed me to get in touch with my anger, the hardest part of my experience with her death. I was angry, but I didn't know where to direct my anger. Was I supposed to be angry with Francesca for having chosen alternative methods? Should I be angry with myself because of something I didn't do? Should I be angry with God? How *do* you get angry with God? It was an abstract concept for me. The play conveniently enough facilitated my rage and allowed me to vent the feelings that were bottled up inside.

It was on opening night that I came to understand another lesson in grief. I stood outside the Powerhouse with the rest of the cast and gazed at Francesca's garden. The producer of the play brought an orange tree to be planted in her memory. There was a small orange blossom on it. We all stood in a circle and held hands in silent reverie. As I looked around, the circle evoked the image of an onion and its different layers. I understood that I had completed one whole cycle in my grief process, one layer of the onion skin, and was now free to move on. I grasped that the next day would not be dramatically different and that passing the one-year mark didn't mean everything would instantly change. Grief doesn't end, it just changes. Francesca was simply receding toward the edge of my consciousness. Like a pebble dropped into a still pond, the rings of her memory were moving outward from the impact point. As my friends spoke of their memories of her, my eyes went to the little blossom and recalled Francesca's love of nature. In the familiar gentle breeze, her voice whispered to me, "Live, Paul, it's okay. Let go and live."

It was fortunate that Chex and I started to deal with our grief before she passed away. Many people suppress their feelings and hope that if they're tough enough, the difficult emotions will pass with time. However, like a submarine lurking in dark waters, these emotions will almost certainly surface at some later point. I learned this firsthand when my dear friend Sal called from New York shortly before Francesca died to find out how things were going with us. Sal, an old college mate and Ryan's godfather, knew about Francesca's breast cancer, but had no idea how grave the situation was.

"How's it going, Papa?" he said. When I explained what was going on, he got upset and wanted to fly right out. I asked him to wait. I already had plenty of help at the time and explained that I would really need him later on, after she died, to help with the children.

Sal lost his mother when he was nine years old, and I figured that his experience would enable him to help my children cope with their own mother's death.

About forty-eight hours later, the phone rang. It was a deeply disturbed Sal. "You know, Paul, when I heard the news the other day, I didn't really get it. You want me to come out and help the kids come to terms with losing their mother. But I have to tell you that since I hung up the phone, I have been so depressed. I feel like I'm having a nervous breakdown."

I listened as he continued. "Paul, even though I told you I'd come, there is no way that I can be of assistance. I realize now that I've never dealt with my own mother's death."

Sal recalled that his dad, in perhaps some classic Italian machismo/denial response to losing his wife, had gotten the kids together the day after her death, taken all the photos and memorabilia that had anything to do with her, and thrown them out. His dad basically said, "Your mom's gone. We will speak of her no more."

Sal had kept those feelings bottled up inside of him for a lifetime. The news of Chex's impending death had triggered this pain to surge to the surface for the first time in many years, and he was overwhelmed by it.

I suggested that maybe Francesca was providing an opportunity for him to bring up these memories for the purpose of healing them. For over twenty-five years, Sal's wound had festered and he had developed substantial emotional scar tissue. To this day, he still struggles to deal with his grief and his fear of abandonment.

A few weeks after Chex's death, I attended my twentieth high school reunion with my closest friend from the class of 1966. He and his wife felt it would be good for me to get out and see some old friends. (Of course, I hadn't liked most of the people back then, and I discovered that two decades hadn't changed anything.) Whenever I encountered a familiar face, the small talk always led to the difficult question, "So, Paul, what's new with you?"

"Well," I replied. "My wife just died and I'm struggling right now." My truthful response ended any further conversation, and I ended up spending the remainder of my reunion sitting with Alan and Beth at a darkened corner table. It hurt me that no one was either willing or able to deal with what I was going through.

The way people would acknowledge my loss also fascinated me. "I know just what you're going through" was a familiar refrain. "I lost my mom," "I lost my best friend," or "I'm going through a divorce." It stunned me that people were so quick to equate losses. Losing a parent in his or her later seventies is a painful part of the natural order. However, it's not the same as losing one's mate, and divorce is a whole other ball game.

One of the main lessons that I gleaned from losing Chex is the importance of acknowledging someone's grief. Many of my friends struggled over whether they should mention Francesca or not. Their desire not to cause me any further pain isolated me. Now I always express my sympathy at another person's loss, in order to give him or her an opportunity to talk about it.

Grief is an individual passage in which there is neither a right nor wrong way. It is an undeniable ritual that needs to be honored and completed. Like a snake shedding its skin, it is a tangible event. Ironically, this painful process is also the means by which healing, catharsis, and spiritual renewal are attained. But this can only happen if one chooses to embrace the experience from that point of view. Otherwise, it can be a disabling and life-negating episode.

"Just let her go" was another verbal panacea frequently expressed to me. But "letting go" of a life partner after ten years is not a simple thing. You don't amputate a person's presence from your existence. She is part of you on a cellular level. Real letting go requires "deep tissue" emotional work—the kind that requires time, courage, and the willingness to open oneself to life again.

The Mother's Day Card

"Jasper, honey...what is that male figure doing?"
"Paul, he's pulling his heart back together."

Two years after Francesca had left us, I was seeing a woman who had become close to the kids. Jasper, then eight years old, had made her a Mother's Day card. A wonderful artist, he'd taken a little piece of pink paper, folded it in half, and had drawn heart-shaped balloons with strings. In the middle of the rising balloon forms was a big heart that had broken into two equal halves. Each half reflected the facets of the break and in between was a little male figure floating in space. The figure's fingertips reached out toward each heart half. The card read, "Even though you're not my mom, I still love you. Happy Mother's Day."

I looked at him and said, "Jasper, honey, tell me. What is that male figure doing on the front of the card between those two heart halves like that?"

I was a forty-year-old man about to get a basic primer in love from an eight-year-old child. A lesson in letting go, in allowing new love to flow in; a lesson in acceptance and moving on, the bottom-line principle of forgiveness. I listened to his answer, amazed that my little boy could so simply understand such a complex issue.

He smiled and said, "Paul, he's pulling his heart back together."

157

Responsibility and Illness

"What did I do? Am I being punished?"

A re we what we eat? Do we create our own reality? Are we responsible for our diseases?

Francesca struggled to come to terms with the idea that she had somehow created her illness. She grappled with the dynamics of fate and free will. Chex examined all the minute details of her past in order to discern what she might have done to manifest her cancer: unexpressed anger, subjugated needs, and guarded fears.

Was she *that* out of touch? Was she a bad person? Was God punishing her for something? What did she do to bring this on? Her guilt was a mighty burden to bear. Did her inability to turn her disease around mean that she was unable or unwilling to get well? Was she choosing to die or was death simply her next dance partner? As if being sick wasn't enough, she also beat herself up for somehow having caused the problem.

Chex visited with spiritualists and spent endless hours listening to tapes recorded during these sessions. She was determined to discern the essence of her responsibility to her illness. Her final determination of liability was split between unexpressed anger and her penchant for spoonfuls of caramelized Thanksgiving turkey scrapings.

One year after Francesca's death, I attended a performance of Joe Kogel's *Life and Depth*, a one-man show about his surviving a particularly fatal type of cancer. During the lively discussion period afterward, a well-dressed older, organic-health-food-type couple expounded on the reality that we are all responsible for our illnesses. I was furious that these two people, who both looked as if they had never been sick a day in their lives, could take such a point of view.

I explained how my late wife had died at age thirty-seven of breast cancer and had suffered greatly in her self-examination of what she could have possibly done to bring this upon herself, her husband, and her kids. My angry response was interrupted by a calming voice who offered a new definition for the word *responsibility:* one's ability to respond.

This new understanding helped me to see that Chex had demonstrated real responsibility in her fight to survive and had done so in the most human way possible.

Macho Man

"If it had been my wife..."

One of the most unexpected responses to my one-man performance of *Time Flies When You're Alive* has been what I now refer to as the Macho Man Response, the archetypal caveman attitude that I *should* (don't you love that word!) have forced Francesca to undergo chemotherapy.

This opinion was first expressed to me at the paddle tennis courts on southern California's Venice Beach. My singles opponent, Mike, and I were lacing up our shoes one morning when he said, "Paul, I have to tell you. I've really been pissed off at you."

"What did I do?" I asked. "Did I give you a bad line call the last time we played?"

"No," he replied. "Ever since I saw your show, I've been thinking about your wife and I've been angry at you. How could you have let her be so foolish?"

"What do you mean?" I pressed. I was totally thrown by the depth of his emotional outburst that followed.

"I can't believe you didn't make her follow the doctor's orders. Let me tell you, if it had been my wife, I would have physically dragged her to his office and forced the medicine down her throat."

"Mike," I replied. "It's just not who we were to one another. Let's play."

161

This same viewpoint was represented by a Paramount Pictures executive who was so angry that he refused to shake my hand after a performance.

I've thought long and hard about this and have come to a few conclusions. First, and most important, Chex did what she believed would get her well. Since it was *her* body, it had to be her choice. She wrestled with her options before taking a path that was right for *her*.

My duty as her husband was to support her in these decisions. Whether I agreed with her or not was never the issue. On our wedding day, I vowed to encourage her fulfillment as an individual, and our relationship had always been based on mutual respect. I believed in her.

In hindsight, it's easy to say that she was wrong and to assume that chemotherapy would have worked. However, it's not that simple. "Following the doctor's orders" is a very naive approach to catastrophic illness and doesn't always result in someone's well-being.

During Francesca's illness, I met a lawyer whose own wife was battling breast cancer. His wife followed doctor's orders to the tee and did all the chemo and radiation prescribed. She even supplemented her program with alternative methods. But her cancer came back. She suffered through a second year of chemotherapy only to die ten and a half months after Francesca. There are no easy solutions when you are battling cancer.

Some people do chemotherapy and live, some people do chemotherapy and die. Some people get well eating brown rice.

Studies have been done to ascertain what various cancer survivors might have in common. *Cancer Survivors* was Francesca's favorite book on the subject because it reinforced her belief that recovery was based on a strong will to live and a positive attitude toward treatment.

Of course, there is the other side of the coin. If we had to go through it all over again, I know I would insist on an immediate

162

evaluation and removal of the lump. That's where we made our mistake. I believe that the reason her breast cancer became fatal was directly due to the one year that her tumor went unchecked. I strongly doubt that the final outcome would have been any different if she'd had chemical therapy.

Years later, I had the opportunity to meet Dr. Decklin Walsh, a world-class oncologist, at the Cleveland Clinic and asked him about cancer of the breast and chemotherapy. He told me that as far as he was concerned, the two greatest weapons against cancer were still *early* detection and surgery.

During her two years of illness, she enjoyed a quality of life superior to that of a typical chemo patient's. Her days were relatively free of pain and side effects, and I was the fortunate beneficiary of her method of treatment.

If I failed at all, it was in not helping her to *react* quickly enough to the problem. In all other ways, I feel that I fulfilled my role as her life mate. Perhaps some people perceived of my actions as merely sitting back and doing nothing. But the fact is, her methods required more effort and participation from me than if I'd coerced her into the traditional route. And what if I had forced her to be a reluctant recipient of chemotherapy, watched her lose her hair, suffer terribly from toxic side effects, and then die? How could I have lived with that? I have no regrets. Just memories.

I do not personally believe that Chex's story is about cancer or chemotherapy. It is about the illusion of control under which we all live. Life is so fragile, yet we choose to forget how delicate the balance really is between life and death. Every person must make his or her own choices. And live with them. God forbid that anyone you know or love should be forced to make these decisions.

Love After Loss

"Papa, when are we going to get a new mom?"
"I'd like you to meet Christine."

I had never expected my life to be invaded by catastrophic illness, nor did I ever imagine that I'd be a single parent at age thirty-seven who was responsible for three small children. But there I was. Mr. Mom. A widower juggling a household, a career, and a desire to start my new life.

During Francesca's dying days, we often talked about my life after she was gone. She wanted me to move on and start living again. She only made two requests: (1) Don't marry for lust, but lust could certainly be a part of the package, however. (2) Only marry someone who loves the kids as much as she loves you. She said, "Paul, I want you to have a lot of hot action after I'm gone. You deserve it after all this cancer stuff."

Finding the next Ms. Right was no easy feat. I was lonely, but unlike so many other widowers, I couldn't jump right back into marriage. Chex and I had been in total sync. We were simpatico. I would wait for the right love.

As far as dating went, I felt like a kid in the candy store. Of course, I was aware of AIDS, herpes, and other factors, but I was not prepared for how much dating had changed. While fantasizing about high-tech "Dick Tracy" radio-watch types of disease detectors (which I called the "dick tracer"), I was forced to confront dating in the late eighties, when foamy café au laits were the only true form of *safe sex*!

165

My initial foray into intimacy was with a woman who insisted on a "no strings attached" relationship, but wanted me to tie her up. I wasn't opposed to either idea—I just lacked the four-poster bed required for the latter. There's more to bondage than one would think. I had lots of old neckties, but nothing to tether them to.

The first time we made love, I found myself checking her breasts for lumps. I wondered if she knew what I was doing and asked myself esoteric questions like: "How long do you see someone before you ask her to have a mammogram? When do you ask her to get a Pap smear? Should we spend our honeymoon at the Mayo Clinic?"

She taught me what I call "turbo sex." I learned that there's sex and then there's turbo sex (a fifth gear of sexuality). About the third or fourth time, she wanted to teach me about tantric sex. It had something to do with my lingam and her yoni—sort of a cosmic sexual smoothie. I didn't fully grasp it, but it was great.

My "no strings attached lover" made it clear from the very start that she had no expectations and simply wanted to go with the flow. I told her that I wasn't ready for a relationship either.

When she wanted to spend the night, I insisted that she sleep in another bedroom. It was important for the kids to find me alone in the bed that I'd occupied with their mother. Until I was serious about someone, I didn't want to upset them by usurping Chex's place. I also felt it was necessary to set a proper moral tone.

After her first sleepover, we dropped the kids off at school and stopped at a local café for croissants and cappuccinos. We ran into an old friend of mine. She was a woman whom I hadn't seen in a long time, and we were happy to connect again.

On the way home, my "no strings attached" lover tearfully confessed that she was in love with me and wanted to be a mother to my children. Seeing me with the "other" woman had been very painful for her. She confided, "Paul, why is it that I always lose good men like you to women like that? I know you want to go out with her. I know it."

I was speechless and tried to keep my eyes on the road.

By the time we parked in front of my house, she was sobbing uncontrollably.

What happened to going with the flow? I thought to myself. What about no strings attached?

As I comforted her, I realized that people are not Legos and that you can't just replug into a relationship. I reached into the backseat of my car and handed her my copy of *The Road Less Traveled*. When it didn't do anything to alleviate her tears, I suggested therapy and pulled out a copy of *Men Who Hate Women and the Women Who Love Them*.

The fact is, she was right. I *did* want to go out with "the other woman."

My "other woman" was a divorcée with two little children who had joie de vivre up the kazoo. We got together with all of our kids and let them run freely on the beach while we held hands and had adult talk. I called her Z. She called me P.

I told her about a dream I'd had. I saw the two of us standing on an enormous grass area, holding each other's hands and looking lovingly into one another's eyes. Our children surrounded us in a circle as they held hands. In a greater ring beyond that, all of our friends encircled us. Everyone was smiling. I felt that the dream signified that my life was moving on and that I was falling in love with her. I told her that I could see spending the rest of my life with her and that my broken heart was mending itself whole.

As I hugged her, I could feel her emotionally and physically pushing me away. Something was wrong.

"Paul, I should have told you this before we started spending so much time together....I have a boyfriend. I love the way you talk about your feelings and truly admire your openness. Even though my boyfriend never tells me anything, and is totally closed off emotionally...and even though he's still married and in a bitter custody battle...I'm going to try to make it work with him."

This revelation left me reeling, and I went home to try and come to terms with this whole notion of "the boyfriend in the closet." My first two relationship attempts had failed. The only thing they had in common was that they were totally opposite. My first lover wanted it and I didn't; in the second, I wanted it, but she didn't. It made me realize that when I lost Francesca, I had also lost someone who totally understood me and shared the same emotional subtext. When I said "A," Chex understood it to mean "A." But now I was in a whole new world where "A" could be "B."

I didn't have time to wallow in self-pity. I had three little children for whom I was responsible. The only person who helped me through this was my El Salvadoran housekeeper. She spoke no English and I spoke what I called actor Spanish. I added an *a* or an *o* to everything and gestured a lot. It was a brutal time. I remember sitting at a tee-ball game with my good friend Dennis and discussing household concerns.

"Dennis," I said. "I need someone who speaks English and drives."

"You mean a wife," he replied sardonically.

I was determined to find love again. But love had taken on a new definition. It now meant finding a wife and a mother. During my first year as a widower, every time I found a seemingly unattached, age-appropriate woman, there were always boyfriends lurking in the closet, ex-husbands with child visitation rights, or simply a lot of excess emotional baggage. Some of these women were dragging around steamer trunks filled with problems and issues. One practically needed a porter to date these women.

Every time I felt a gentle breeze, I thought back on the moment that Chex died. I remember thinking that my experience with her had taught me exactly what love meant. Love was the end result of the process. It entailed going every step of the way with your partner, through the fear of abandonment and fear of commitment, and climbing every rung together. Love was the by-product of all this effort. I thought I had achieved a knowledge that I would take with me throughout my life. It would enable me to create relationships and make love happen again. However, the truth was I couldn't find the right woman with whom to share my hard-earned knowledge.

I don't understand why you can't ever find someone when you're looking for her. It's a phenomenon that defies explanation, but it's always been true for me. The minute you stop looking, she's there. I've often wondered if pretending you're not looking would work.

There was a huge hole in my life. The kids had their needs, and I had mine too. I knew I was in trouble when I dreamed of merging those needs by finding the perfect nanny who might also be willing to sleep with me.

Finally, I gave up, and of course, as soon as I did, I met someone. A tall blond older woman who was Swedish. We were two Tauruses in a hot steamy kitchen at a party in Santa Monica. We immediately connected and began to date.

I had just terminated a "nanny from hell" who had a drug problem and had disappeared with my car for three days. In these circumstances, our relationship catapulted forward and within a year she'd become like a wife and mother.

My new therapist, Allan Rosenthal, broached the issue of our relationship and my intentions.

"Well," he said to me, "have you decided what you want to do?"

I hated whenever a therapist asked a question in such a way that implied the answer was obvious to everyone else but me. He recognized the ambivalence in my heart. A part of me loved how she was with the kids and I hoped this would lead me to fall in love with her. But the other part of me believed that she was not the right person. No emotional subtext existed between us. She was content with the fact that we were compatible, but frankly, there has to be more to life than both parties wanting chicken for dinner.

I'd thought the *A* word for dating in the eighties and nineties was AIDS. For me it was ambivalence and it was painful.

This internal war raged within me for two years. During that time, we repeated the pattern of breaking up, getting back together, and breaking up. She wanted marriage. I remained uncertain. Finally, she issued an ultimatum to marry her or else, but I couldn't go through with it.

The night we broke up for good, I went to see how the kids were doing. Jasper was crying.

"Jasper, honey, listen. I know how much you love her. And I know you wanted her to be your mom. But you must understand…you see, unless you have a very special feeling in your heart for someone, you shouldn't marry them. As much as I know you would have liked me to, this is one thing I can't do for you."

Sadly, he looked at me and said, "But Paul, what if you never have that special feeling again?"

"I will, Jasper. I know I will."

Rosie threw in her two cents by adding, "Papa, when are we going to get a new mom?"

"Well, Rosie, I don't know, honey. Do you want one?"

"Yes, I do."

"Rosie, what kind of a mom do you want?"

"Anyone you can find."

In the aftermath of my failed December-May romance, I directed all of my energy into my work and my children. Four years had passed since Francesca had died. Finally, I began to feel as though my life was back on track. I decided that if I ever had another relationship, it would be one based on choice and not need. I would no longer look.

My life truly began again on May 31, 1990.

"I'd like you to meet Christine Healy." My friend Kate Mulgrew said these words to me as she stood next to a shapely, beautiful, blue-eyed brunette. We were at an opening night party for the Mark Taper Forum's production of *Aristocrats* by Brian Friel in which they both were appearing. I didn't realize it at the time, but Kate was doing some serious matchmaking. It was a setup, but no one had told me. Christine wore a white silk evening pantsuit, and when she smiled, the room filled with light. As Christine and I shook hands, a photographer appeared and snapped our picture. As it turns out, this photo captured a most important moment in both of our lives. Kismet.

Kate's instincts were correct. We were perfect for each other and the conversation flowed easily. It felt so comfortable, so right. We talked until the restaurant closed. When I got home, I immediately called to make sure that she'd gotten home safely.

Christine had never been married, nor had any children. She was an accomplished actress in regional theater who had supported herself for fifteen years before moving to Los Angeles for television and film work. A middle child born in Buffalo, New York, she was the daughter of former sportscaster Chuck Healy and his wife, Jean.

We had two dates before I headed off to Dallas for two months to appear in Elizabeth Forsythe Hailey's stage version of *Joanna's Husband, David's Wife*. The beginning of our relationship was forged in letters, cards, and two-hour, late-night phone calls. Our romance blossomed the old-fashioned way...we earned it.

As soon as I returned home, Christine and I began our courtship. From the very start, she brought laughter and sweetness into my life. Through her, I discovered that what I'd felt had been lacking in my life truly existed. I had given up hope, but there she was with all the qualities and emotional subtext that I'd been longing for.

Our intentions were serious from the very beginning. She started to visit the house and get to know the children. Christine approached her relationship with Jasper, Ryan, and Rose with responsibility and respect. I admired her concerns about entering the children's life prematurely. We recognized their need for a mother, and neither one of us wanted to disappoint them. Until we were certain about our own future together, we didn't want her to take on too important a role in their lives.

We moved slowly, one drawer at a time, but it didn't take long before Christine spent all of her time with us. Christine filled me with happiness and brought a gentle kindness to Michael Avenue. The kids absolutely adored her and she them. By Christmas it was clear that I loved her and that she was the person with whom I wanted to spend my life. She was the first person whom I felt good about my children calling Mom.

On February 1, 1991, I asked Christine to be my wife. I'd had great fantasies about the moment, and all sorts of plans had flashed through my mind. The actual milestone, however, took place at the breakfast table over coffee. As I sat there in my horrible, multicolored terry cloth robe, reading the sports page, I hurled myself to my knees, extended my hand to her across the *Los Angeles Times* which was spread in front of me, and proposed.

"Will you marry me?"

Taking on a husband and three children was not a trivial decision. She was giving up a lot, but gaining a great deal too. One week later, she said yes.

June 15, 1991. We gathered with our family and friends in a glen of oak trees nestled in the mountains high above Malibu. A former Indian village, the grounds where the ceremony was performed were considered sacred. Beneath a brilliant blue sky, we pledged our vows. Jasper and his friends Jason and Michael sang a Shaker hymn. When their sweet young voices filled the air, tears flowed and hearts burst. Christine and I each took a moment to express our feelings. Her sentiments were eloquent and from such a deep place within her soul that the words overwhelmed me. I realized, as I told her, I was no longer a "one-man show." When we were pronounced husband and wife, the children encircled us as we kissed. I had finally completed my passage through loss to love.

My beautiful bride has made my life as full and happy as it has ever been. She nurtures our children and has helped teach me the way back into my own heart. I'm so lucky to have found love again. And there's lots of lust in the deal.

One time Christine had to go away to a film location. Six-year-old Rosie was very nervous about the impending departure. To help relieve Rosie's "separation anxiety," Christine bought her a heart-shaped locket into which a small picture could be inserted.

There is a photograph, taken at Thanksgiving 1990, of Christine, me, and the three children. We are sitting on a bright orange couch, our bodies all intertwined with one another, and our faces are absolutely beaming with joy. We call it "the happy family photo."

She selected one of the many copies we had reproduced and cut out only her face, leaving the rest of the picture intact. Rose sat on the bed with her and assisted in the operation. She picked up the cut-up photo, which now had an empty heart-shaped space where Christine's face had been. She studied it for a long time and stated with utter simplicity, "Before you came, we were just half a family, waiting for someone to fill in the heart."

TIME FLIES WHEN YOU'RE ALIVE

About the Author

Paul Linke, a professional actor for almost twenty years and best known for his role as Artie Grossman in the television series "CHiPs," first presented this story as a monologue by the same name in Los Angeles, where it played for over a year. The play then went on to San Francisco, Seattle, Dallas, Santa Fe, Detroit, Philadelphia, and ultimately to Off Broadway. It was also a critically acclaimed HBO film. Linke subsequently remarried and lives in Los Angeles with his wife, actress Christine Healy, and his children. They are expecting a baby girl in early 1993.